The Fertility Kitchen

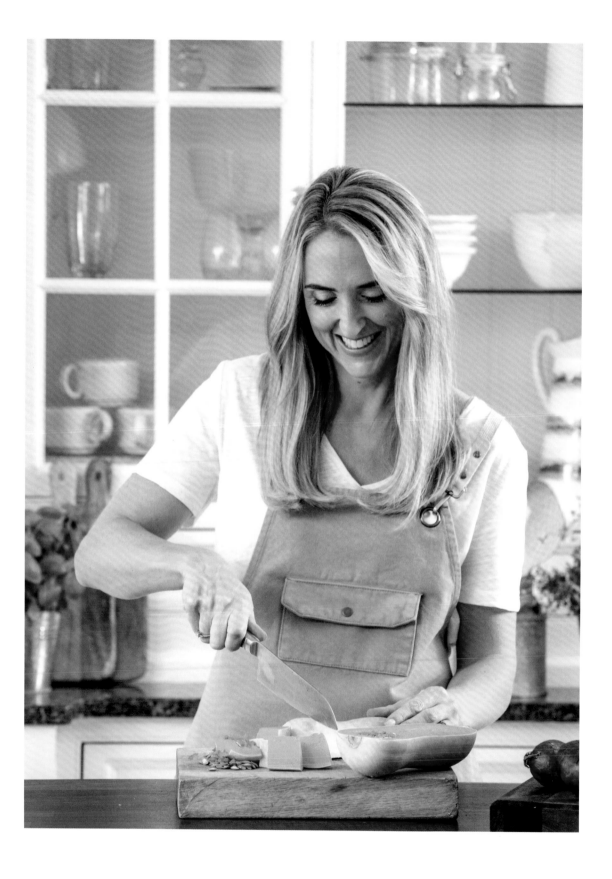

Charlotte Grand

The Fertility Kitchen

The essential guide to supporting your fertility

QUERCUS

For my boys. I love you more than my whole life.

First published in Great Britain in 2022 by

Quercus Editions Ltd
Carmelite House
50 Victoria Embankment
London EC4Y 0DZ

An Hachette UK company

A CIP catalogue record for this book is available from the British Library

ISBN 978 1 52941 721 0

10 9 8 7 6 5 4 3 2 1

Designed and typeset by Tokiko Morishima
Copy editor: Corinne Colvin
Photographer: Andrew Hayes-Watkins
Food stylists: Ellie Mulligan, Charlotte Grand
Props stylist: Charlotte Grand
Illustrator: Peter Liddiard
Proofreader: Anna Southgate

Printed and bound in China by C&C Offset Printing Co., Ltd.

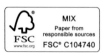

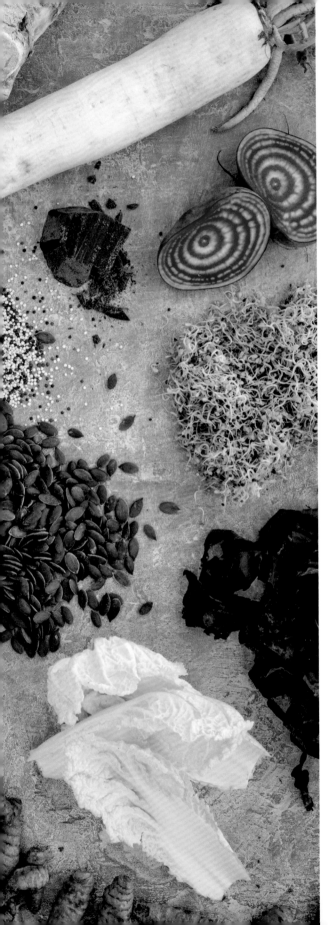

Contents

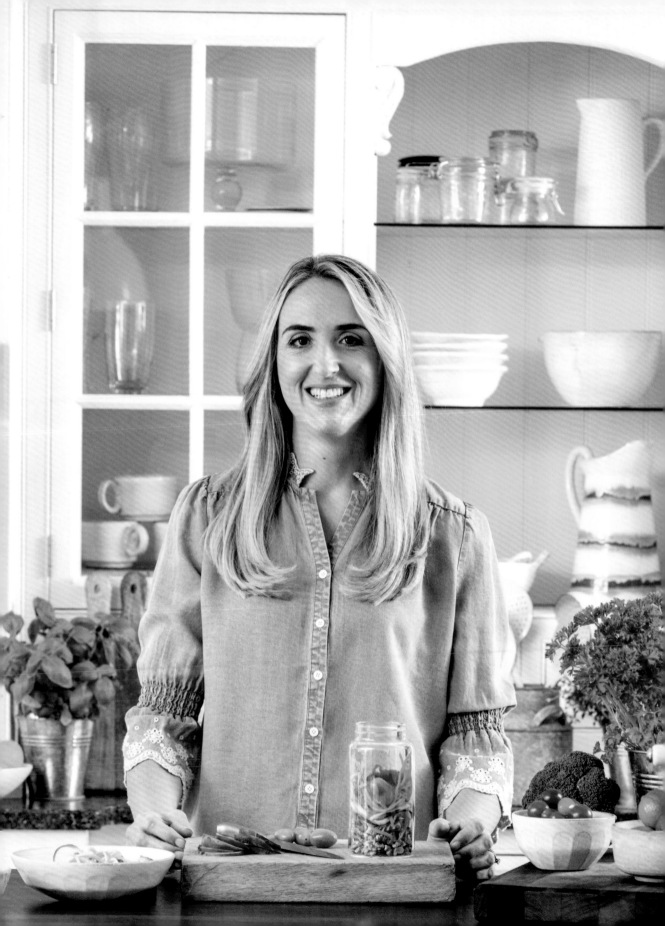

Welcome to The Fertility Kitchen

My story

Hi, I'm Charlotte. Thank you for picking up this book; I know that you've found me at the right stage of your fertility journey. I've written this book to help you get actively involved in your fertility healthcare.

Back in 2008, I was struggling to conceive my first child. I'd spent most of my adult life trying not to get pregnant, so when we wanted a baby I (naively) assumed it would happen straight away, or at least while we were still having fun trying!

I had a textbook menstrual cycle and we were both young, fit and healthy. On paper it should have happened easily. Fast forward three long years and we were embarking on IVF after being diagnosed with unexplained infertility. This wasn't how I'd envisaged conceiving our baby.

I'd seen countless friends get pregnant at lightning speed. Undoubtedly the hardest part of infertility was watching friends welcome their second baby into the world while we were still trying for our first. I felt so sad and lived with a deep sense of longing. This spurred me into action, and I became determined to learn how to nourish my body to give us the best chance of conception.

Firstly, I sought acupuncture treatment (a rite of passage when trying to conceive?!) to help with the stress of it all. I still vividly remember my astonishment at my first pain-free period after years of monthly agony. How could a few needles have such a profound effect? I began to research Chinese medicine and I loved it; the approach to healing resonated and I wanted in. Cutting a long story short, I left my career in the fashion world to retrain in acupuncture. I've never looked back.

Shortly after I started acupuncture training, I began preparing for IVF. My nutrition knowledge was basic, so I researched how to use diet and lifestyle to support treatment. It was difficult to find practical advice; I found information on the benefits of specific nutrients, but nothing transforming this into real food and everyday eating. So, I started creating my own recipes, incorporating everything my research suggested I needed. My first creation was a protein smoothie that I drank everyday throughout IVF.

I also slowly upgraded my day-to-day lifestyle, incorporating practices to nourish my mind and body as much as possible. As well as acupuncture, I exercised and meditated daily, used positive affirmations, kept a gratitude journal and prioritised sleep. These practices attenuated my stress levels, and I felt incredible despite navigating IVF. We were blessed to conceive our son, George.

After qualifying I set up a fertility acupuncture clinic and through my work, observed a strong connection between diet, lifestyle and fertility. After the birth of my second son, Alex, I continued exploring how to optimise my own health. Over time I completely overhauled my diet, experiencing first-hand the power of food as medicine; most pertinently the asthma I'd suffered with since childhood resolved. It was a defining moment that changed my trajectory and I embarked on extensive training in the field of nutritional therapy, completing a three-year diploma at the Institute for Optimum Nutrition in Richmond.

Meanwhile, I continued writing recipes. This reignited my creativity, which I'd missed since leaving fashion. I've always had a great passion for cooking (and eating!) and saw an opportunity to combine my love of food and creative flare through recipe writing, food styling and photography, with a newfound passion for helping women to take ownership of their fertility.

One morning I sat reflecting on my journey. I'd come to realise that my experience wasn't unique and other women were also dissatisfied with the lack of fertility nutrition and lifestyle advice available. I thought about how I could draw on my personal and professional experience to educate and inspire others and create a community for women on their path to motherhood. I had a lightbulb moment, and The Fertility Kitchen was born.

The three pillars

My guiding philosophy embodies my vision for The Fertility Kitchen and sits at the heart of everything I do. It extends beyond food and nutrition to encompass the entire framework of lifestyle and wellbeing and is built on three pillars: Fertility, Food and Life.

Fertility
Empowerment underpins the Fertility pillar. Here I share how to create a personalised nutrition and lifestyle plan. The Fertility pillar covers six foundations for optimal health and fertility (gut health, blood-sugar balance, liver detoxification, thyroid health, egg quality and your partner's sperm quality), helps you identify any issues in these areas and support them through Food and Life.

Food
Food provides the building blocks for new cells, so a preconception diet quite literally lays the foundations of your future child's health. This inspires the Food pillar, which combines evidence-based nutrition information, alongside the practical advice and whole-food recipes needed to implement it. This will help you find a sustainable and balanced approach to eating for your fertility and for life.

Life
The Life pillar demonstrates how optimal fertility also relies upon a healthy lifestyle that nourishes your complete wellbeing. This encompasses stress, sleep, movement, environment and mindset. I encourage you to determine which factors you need to bring into balance and what you can do to help yourself in these areas.

The first half of this book takes you through the three pillars; the second half is dedicated to the recipes. Each pillar is connected and the recommendations in Fertility naturally lead into Food and Life. By combining these elements, you will be able to create a diet and lifestyle that supports your fertility and provides your future child with the best opportunity to thrive.

This is the guide that I needed on my journey, and I hope it supports you on yours.

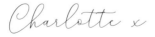

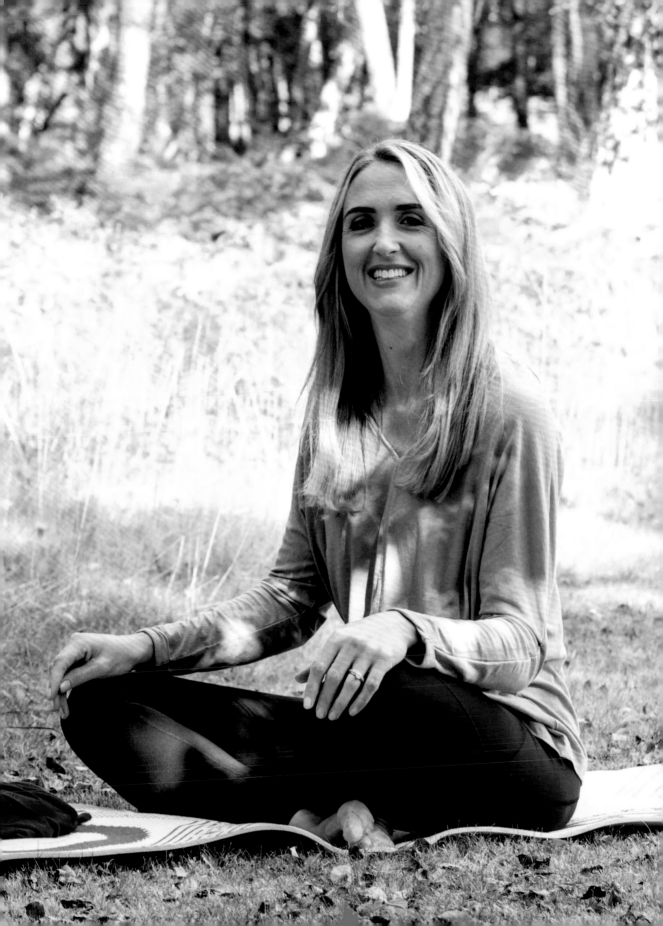

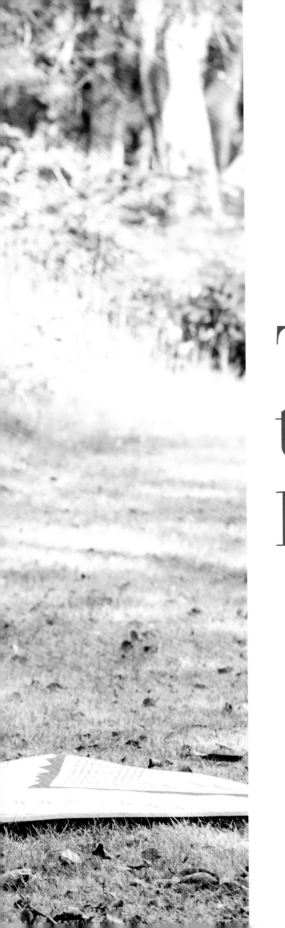

The three pillars

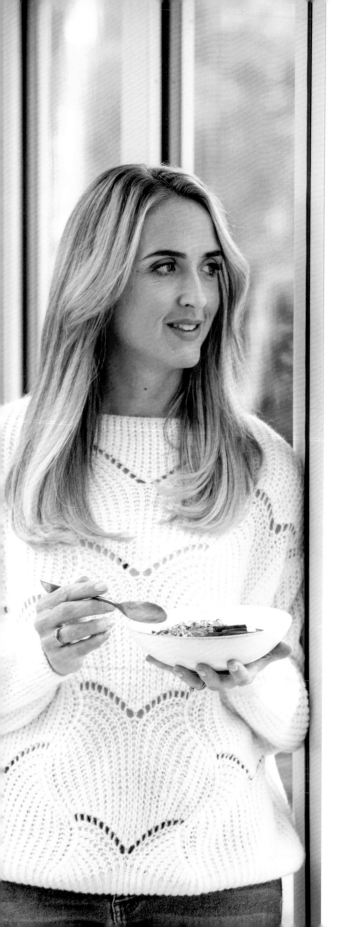

Fertility

When you think about supporting your fertility you may be focused on your reproductive system because you are used to the idea that individual body systems can be treated in isolation. However, our bodies are far more complex, and multiple systems work together for healthy fertility. Your gut health, state of inflammation and autoimmunity, blood-sugar balance, liver function and detoxification, thyroid function and egg quality, and your partner's sperm quality, are factors that can profoundly impact your ability to conceive and enjoy a healthy pregnancy.

Start with your gut

Gut health is central to overall health. Your body depends on a healthy gut function for nutrient absorption, healthy immune function, hormonal balance and detoxification.

Digestion basics

Optimal digestion is vital for absorbing nutrients from your food, which in turn are essential for supporting fertility and a healthy pregnancy. If you're not digesting and absorbing well, it really doesn't matter how healthy your diet is – it's unlikely that you'll be getting the nutrients required to fully support your fertility.

Digestion begins in your brain. Thinking about food and experiencing it through sight and smell prepares you for digestion – your mouth waters as you anticipate your meal. Chewing your food thoroughly mechanically breaks it down and releases salivary amylase to begin starch digestion.

When food reaches your stomach, stomach acid (HCl) and pepsin begin protein digestion and separate essential nutrients for absorption in the small intestine. Low stomach acid is a common issue because stress, refined carbohydrates, medications (proton pump inhibitors (PPIs), non-steroidal anti-inflammatory drugs (NSAIDs), the contraceptive pill), nutrient deficiencies, food sensitivities and alcohol can deplete it. You also need optimal HCl levels to trigger the next stage of digestion, which moves food into the small intestine. If you eat when feeling stressed or anxious you may notice a feeling of fullness, bloating or heartburn as the food begins to ferment in your tummy.

When food reaches your small intestine, your pancreas releases bicarbonate and pancreatic enzymes to neutralise stomach acid and prepare nutrients for absorption. Your gallbladder releases bile to emulsify fats. Leftovers, such as fibre and other waste, become food for your gut bacteria in the colon. Gut bacteria ferment fibre and produce nutrients such as short-chain fatty acids, B vitamins and vitamin K_2 to keep the cells of the colon healthy. Bacteria also help move waste through the colon for excretion. Since there are multiple steps and organs involved in the digestive process, there are many potential opportunities for issues to arise.

Stress and digestion

Optimal digestion relies on you being in a relaxed state. Stress and anxiety shift you into fight or flight; in this state your body prioritises survival, and digestion will be put on the back burner. The stress response can be triggered in a single instant, so it's not ideal to eat while working, looking at your phone, watching TV, or if you're feeling anxious. Habits I think we're all guilty of!

A stressed eater = sympathetic dominance (fight or flight) = digestion OFF

A relaxed eater = parasympathetic dominance (rest and digest) = digestion ON

Intestinal permeability (aka leaky gut)

Your digestive tract is separated from your bloodstream by a thin border made of mucosal cells. These cells are tightly packed together to form a protective barrier between the outside world and inside your body, regulating what's allowed in and out. In order to pass through this barrier, your food must be fully digested into tiny particles.

Increased intestinal permeability (leaky gut) occurs when the tight junctions between these border cells become loose, allowing incompletely digested food molecules, pathogens and waste products to enter the bloodstream. Leaky gut can happen in response to chronic stress, a poor-quality diet, undigested food particles, imbalanced gut bacteria (dysbiosis), infections, toxins and medications, such as NSAIDs and the contraceptive pill.

Since about 70 per cent of your body's immune system is housed in the gut, when larger food molecules and other particles enter the bloodstream, they trigger an inflammatory response. Inflammation is meant to be a short-lived, protective process but becomes an issue when it is chronic and unresolved. Modern living contributes to a state of chronic inflammation as our bodies are constantly dealing with a poor diet and stressful lifestyle.

Chronic Inflammation has been linked to insulin resistance, ovarian dysfunction and polycystic ovary syndrome (PCOS), poor egg quality and impaired ovulation, endometriosis and recurrent miscarriage.

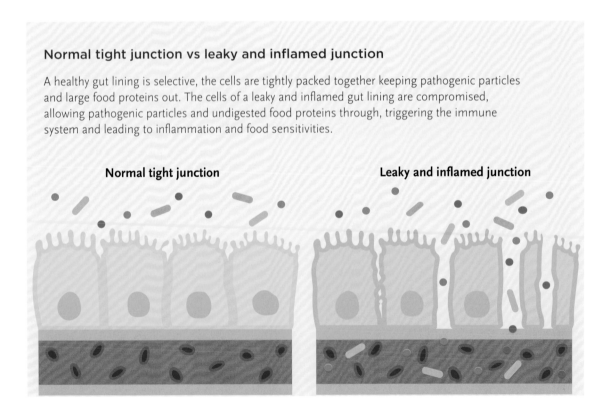

Normal tight junction vs leaky and inflamed junction

A healthy gut lining is selective, the cells are tightly packed together keeping pathogenic particles and large food proteins out. The cells of a leaky and inflamed gut lining are compromised, allowing pathogenic particles and undigested food proteins through, triggering the immune system and leading to inflammation and food sensitivities.

Normal tight junction

Leaky and inflamed junction

Autoimmunity

Autoimmunity is a condition of immune confusion, where the body mistakenly attacks its own healthy tissues. Your immune system is continuously guarding against foreign molecules and when it identifies these, it sends out an army of fighter cells to destroy them. Sometimes this goes wrong, and instead of targeting foreign molecules, healthy tissues and hormones become the focus of attack.

A leaky gut, genetics and a triggering event provide the perfect storm for autoimmunity to develop. A leaky gut allows foreign proteins to enter the bloodstream and since most of your immune system is housed in your gut, it's a prime location to trigger immune confusion. Next, you must have the genetic blueprint that puts you at risk. Finally, a triggering event challenges your immune system and increases the likelihood that it will make a mistake. Common triggers include food sensitivities, infections, parasites, chronic stress, toxins, medications and pregnancy.

Autoimmunity can manifest as infertility or pregnancy loss. Autoimmune conditions such as systemic lupus erythematosus, anti-phospholipid syndrome, thyroid autoimmunity and coeliac disease are associated with infertility and miscarriage. Antibodies such as antiphospholipid, antithyroid or antinuclear may be directly associated with infertility without obvious symptoms, and autoimmunity may affect all stages of fertility, including ovarian and testicular failure, implantation failure and pregnancy loss.

Endometriosis and PCOS have both been associated with altered immune function and a greater prevalence of autoimmune disease.

The good news is that there is a lot you can do to soothe inflammation, support your gut health, balance hormones and reduce your risk for autoimmunity.

Hormone balance, detoxification and your gut

Your gut houses your microbiome, which consists of trillions of bacteria. There is a strong connection between your gut, your microbiome and hormone health. When hormones have done their job, your body packages them up for safe elimination so they don't continue to act. This is done primarily through the gut. Issues like constipation or an imbalance of gut bacteria (dysbiosis) can prevent your body from properly detoxifying and eliminating hormones, especially oestrogen. This can lead to reabsorption, which may affect hormone balance and cause unpleasant symptoms like bloating, cramping, heavy periods and irritability. It is essential to move your bowels every day to remove the oestrogen your body no longer needs.

Does your gut need some TLC?

Regularly experiencing any of the following symptoms suggests that your gut may require support:

- **Bloating and wind**
- **Discomfort and/or belching after meals**
- **Nausea**
- **Heartburn or acid reflux**
- **Feeling of fullness, food sitting in tummy**
- **Stomach cramps**
- **Diarrhoea or loose stools**
- **Constipation or difficulty passing stools**
- **IBS**
- **Undigested food in stools**
- **Hives, rashes, eczema, acne, rosacea**

- Allergies, asthma, sinus infections, stuffy nose
- Fungus or yeast infections

Associated conditions
- Autoimmune disease (suspected or diagnosed)
- Endometriosis
- PCOS
- Implantation failure
- Recurrent miscarriage
- Unexplained infertility

Optimising gut health

Gut rebalancing takes time but can be transformative. The Institute for Functional Medicine's (IFM) 5R framework helps restore balance through five steps: remove, replace, repopulate, repair and rebalance. You don't have to implement all steps at once, but aim to work through them all.

Remove

The goal is to remove potentially inflammatory foods. Leaky gut and food sensitivities go hand-in-hand, so it's important to remove foods that may cause sensitivity to improve gut health. Food sensitivities can be hard to identify because they can result in a diverse range of symptoms and both immediate and delayed reactions are possible.

Consistently eating foods that you are sensitive to leaves the immune system in a constant state of alarm, resulting in leaky gut and chronic inflammation. You may find that despite your best efforts to improve your health, you still don't manage to conceive. By uncovering food sensitivities, you may dramatically improve your situation.

The most common sensitivities I encounter in clinic are gluten, dairy and soy.

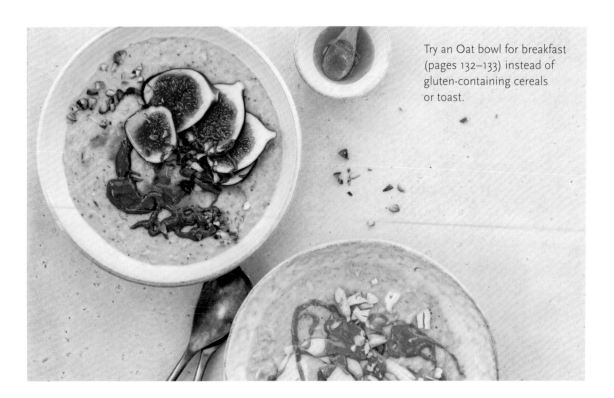

Try an Oat bowl for breakfast (pages 132–133) instead of gluten-containing cereals or toast.

To test for sensitivity, remove each food group completely for at least 30 days. You can remove them altogether, but if this feels too overwhelming, remove one group at a time. Reintroduction is straightforward: add foods within each group back in systematically, each for two to three days at a time. Observe how you feel based on symptoms in the couple of hours after eating the food and over the next two to three days. If you experience any of the symptoms listed above, continue to avoid and repeat in another 30 days. If you feel noticeably better during removal it isn't necessary to reintroduce any of these foods if you don't want to.

Gluten is the protein found in wheat and other grains. Wheat is the most common source of gluten, but gluten is also found in barley, rye, triticale, farina, kamut, spelt, wheat berries, farro and couscous. It can also contaminate oats, so when you avoid gluten make sure you buy gluten-free oats or avoid oats as well. The main sources of gluten are bread, cakes, cereal, condiments, crackers, flour, pasta and pizza. But don't despair – there are many inherently gluten-free, nutrient-rich, whole foods you can replace them with.

Dairy isn't an issue for everyone but can be problematic. Once you have completed the full 30 days removal of dairy, explore what works for you by reintroducing different types of dairy products, one at a time, and note if you experience symptoms. For example, you may experience symptoms from consuming cow's milk but not from yoghurt.

GLUTEN: Swap this for that

BREAD → Seed and nut gluten-free loaf (page 136).

CAKES → Dreamy chocolate tahini brownies (page 214). They are flourless and naturally gluten-free.

CEREAL → Homemade Granola (pages 140–141) Oat bowls (pages 132–133) or eggs (pages 126–130).

CONDIMENTS → As well as gluten, processed condiments tend to be full of sugar. Get rid and choose a delicious dressing (pages 204–207) or make the most of nature's seasonings by using fresh herbs, garlic, olive oil, sea salt and turmeric instead. Soy sauce contains gluten so look for tamari (page 93) instead, or coconut aminos if you're avoiding soy.

CRACKERS → Super-seedy crackers (page 146) or Veggie crisps (page 198).

FLOUR → Ground nuts and seeds, buckwheat, cassava or oat flour (see Pantry staples, pages 82–94).

PASTA → Replace spaghetti and noodles with courgette, sweet potato or squash noodles.

COUSCOUS → Veggie rice (pages 195–197).

PIZZA → Cauliflower pizza base (page 174).

These types of dairy tend to be better tolerated

- **Yoghurt and kefir:** these are more digestible due to the presence of bacteria, which decrease lactose (milk sugar).
- **Goat's milk and yoghurt:** can work for some people who are sensitive to cow's milk.
- **Hard cheeses:** these have a lower lactose content, so can be easier for those with lactose sensitivity to digest. It doesn't help if you are sensitive to milk proteins.
- **Ghee:** this is clarified butter, so does not contain milk protein. You may be able to use this for cooking and spreading (use sparingly, see page 61 – fat section).

If you can tolerate dairy, keep in mind that quality is key and use it as a flavour highlight – think sprinkle rather than slab! Look for non-homogenised whole milk from organic grass-fed cows and avoid low-fat and fat-free, which provide less nutrition and tend to be higher in sugar. Full-fat dairy has been shown to improve fertility, while low-fat dairy may contribute to infertility.

DAIRY: Swap this for that

BUTTER → Flavourless coconut oil for spreading, baking or roasting when you don't want a coconut flavour. Extra virgin coconut oil for when you want the flavour, such as for coconut curry (page 166).

CHEESE → Cashew cheese is easy to make and gives a wonderful creamy texture. Use this in place of cheese sauce (see Creamy cashew dressing on page 204). Nutritional yeast flakes (see Pantry staples on page 91) are great for sprinkling over Bolognese or anything where you'd usually use hard cheese. For something more akin to cow's cheese, look for nut or coconut cheese, but check the ingredients and use sparingly.

MILK → Make your own organic plant milks (page 137). Be wary of boxed supermarket plant milks, which can be sweetened, thickened with gums and contain inflammatory oils to prevent separation. If you do buy boxed, choose organic and unsweetened with minimal ingredients (read the label). My favourite brand is Plenish.

YOGHURT → You can't beat coconut yoghurt: it's thick and creamy and is my go-to topping for homemade Granola (pages 140–141), Oat bowls (pages 132–133), soups (pages 144–147) and curries (pages 166 and 169). My favourite brand is COCOS. Again, read the labels and choose minimal ingredients.

A note on calcium

If you're concerned about meeting your calcium needs while avoiding dairy, then don't worry. Dark-green leafy vegetables, whole sardines (with the bones), sesame seeds and tahini are rich sources. Include plenty of these foods in your diet and you'll have no trouble meeting your needs.

Soy tends to be heavily sprayed with pesticides (unless organic) and contains anti-nutrients (phytic acid and digestive enzyme inhibitors), which may interfere with mineral absorption and protein digestion. Soy may also affect hormone balance and is a common food allergen. If you can tolerate soy, then choose organic, whole soy foods and avoid soybean oil or textured vegetable protein. I recommend organic edamame, tamari and miso used moderately. Traditionally fermented soy products, such as miso, tamari and tempeh, contain less phytic acid due to the fermentation process, so may be better tolerated.

Other common food triggers that may cause sensitivity include corn, eggs, nuts, nightshades (aubergine, bell peppers, potatoes and tomatoes), legumes and yeast. You may wish to experiment with removal and reintroduction of some of these foods if you suspect sensitivity. Food sensitivities can be hard to unearth, so if you're having difficulty establishing what may be an issue for you, seek the support of a nutritional therapist.

Replace

Support gut transit time and motility and include nutrients to optimise digestive secretions:

Eat fibre. Aim for at least 30g of fibre every day. This should be easy to achieve if you make vegetables the foundation of your diet (page 49). Fibre acts as fuel for your gut bacteria. Soluble fibre, found in apples, oats, flaxseeds, chia seeds, psyllium and most vegetables, helps prevent constipation. To increase soluble fibre, try Oat bowls (pages 132–133), Apple pie pancakes (page 124), Seed and nut gluten-free loaf (page 136) and Tiramisu chia puddings (page 221).

SOY: Swap this for that

MILK ➔ DIY plant milks (see page 137) or non-homogenised whole milk from organic grass-fed cows.

SOYBEAN OIL ➔ This is often added to processed foods, so check food labels. If you use this as an oil for cooking, switch to coconut oil (either extra virgin or flavourless), avocado oil, organic grass-fed butter, or ghee or olive oil.

TOFU OR TEMPEH ➔ Use beans and legumes as your protein source if you are vegan.

TAMARI OR SOY SAUCE ➔ Coconut aminos (see Pantry staples on page 86) can directly replace soy sauce and tamari in recipes.

TEXTURED VEGETABLE (SOY) PROTEIN (found in meat substitutes) ➔ Instead of using meat substitutes, try Beetroot burgers (page 177) or use beans and legumes in vegan recipes such as chilli or Bolognese.

YOGHURT ➔ Replace with coconut yoghurt or organic full-fat dairy yoghurt. Avoid low-fat and flavoured yoghurts, which tend to be high in sugar. Instead, add fresh berries to yoghurt for flavour.

Strive for vegetable variety. The magic number for gut diversity is 30+ unique varieties of plants every week. See pages 51–53 for help with this.

Optimise stomach acid (HCl). Zinc is a co-factor for stomach acid production and supports tissue healing and sense of taste. Found in shellfish, meat, eggs and seeds (especially hemp, pumpkin and sesame seeds). Animal sources are superior. Try Yellow coconut curry with tiger prawns (page 166).

Eat naturally bitter foods such as chicory, collard (spring) greens, kale, rocket, spinach and watercress to stimulate your liver to produce bile. Bile acids are critical for the digestion and absorption of fats and fat-soluble vitamins.

Repopulate

Make a happy home for your gut bacteria:

Include prebiotic foods. Prebiotic fibres provide food for beneficial bacteria. Good sources include apples, Jerusalem artichokes, asparagus, garlic, leeks and onions. Try adding artichokes to Green goddess cauliflower pizza (page 174) or a Summer vegetable traybake (page 187).

Eat fermented foods. Fermented foods are abundant in beneficial microbes and prebiotic fibres. Live yoghurt, kefir, kimchi and sauerkraut are all probiotic foods. Make kimchi and sauerkraut yourself, which are easy to make and cheaper than store-bought (pages 191–192).

Repair

Include foods rich in nutrients that help restore the gut lining to optimise nutrient absorption and immune tolerance:

Collagen. Bone broth (stock) is one of the most nourishing foods for the gut. It is

Try this

Easy ways to integrate fermented foods into everyday eating:

- SOUP: add a swirl of kefir or live yoghurt
- SALAD: add a spoonful of sauerkraut or kimchi
- EGGS: spice up scrambled eggs or an omelette with a spoonful of kimchi
- FISH OR MEAT: mix spices into coconut yoghurt to use as a marinade (try Tandoori salmon skewers on page 163).

Smart supplements for gut health

Under the guidance of a nutritional therapist, consider the following:

- BETAINE HCl with pepsin to optimise stomach acid and protein digestion.
- DIGESTIVE ENZYMES to help your body break down food properly.
- OX BILE to support fat digestion, especially if you experience light-coloured, floating or greasy stools, or loose stools after eating a fat-rich meal.
- DIGESTIVE BITTERS to help activate bitter receptors, support bile flow and stimulate healthy digestion.
- PROBIOTIC to support a normal balance of gut bacteria. Look for a combination of Lactobacillus and Bifidobacterium species. Lactobacillus-dominant microbiota have been linked to better IVF outcomes.

rich in collagen, a key protein within the gut lining. Enjoy a daily cup of Boosted stock (page 153). You can also buy collagen (see Resources on page 235) to add to smoothies (pages 138–139) and hot drinks (pages 224–227).

L-glutamine. This amino acid is considered one of the most important nutrients to support gut healing. The best sources of l-glutamine are animal proteins, such as fish, poultry, beef and eggs. Try Lemon-and-herb-crusted roast chicken (page 172), fish recipes (pages 161–164), Slow-cooked beef and black bean chilli (page 168) or egg recipes (pages 126–130).

Omega-3 fatty acids. These fats help reduce inflammation and improve gut health. You'll find them most abundantly in oily fish (pages 148–151 and 163–164).

Vitamin A. Needed for the health of mucosal cells. Eggs and liver are abundant in vitamin A. Find egg inspiration on pages 126–130 and recipes with hidden liver on pages 168 and 178.

Vitamin C. Dark-green leafy vegetables, broccoli, bell peppers and berries are rich in vitamin C, which is needed for collagen synthesis. Eat a plant-centric diet and you'll be getting plenty of vitamin C. Boost intake with Antioxidant burst soft serve (page 218) or A berry good start smoothie (page 139).

Vitamin D. Important for immune function, vitamin D is made in your skin in response to sun exposure. You may need to supplement but check your levels first via your GP or an online blood-testing service (see Resources on page 235). Food sources are eggs, liver, oily fish and red meat.

Rebalance

This is possibly the hardest step as it involves breaking habits and managing stress as an underlying cause of digestive distress. Find strategies on pages 99–110 to help address stress and practise mindful eating, which can help you switch from digestive shutdown to full digestive force.

Mindful eating

This is an approach to eating that focuses on bringing your full attention to your food and the experience of eating, moment by moment and without judgment. Try these tips for mindful eating:

- Prepare your food yourself to help build anticipation for the meal ahead and kick off the digestive process.
- When you are eating just eat, even if you step away from work for just 15 minutes.
- Sit at a table, free from distraction.
- Take three to five deep, calming breaths before starting your meal.
- Focus on the sight, smell and taste of your food.
- Chew each mouthful to a purée – 30 chews should do the trick!
- Slow down. Take a break between bites and put your knife and fork down.
- Take pleasure in every bite. Enjoying your food ramps up production of those all-important digestive juices.
- Listen to your body and recognise when you've had enough. We are conditioned to leave our plates clean, but it's not necessary. Leftovers can be saved for another time.
- If you feel very stressed or anxious, consider delaying your meal until you feel calmer.
- Tune into your body's hunger signals. If you notice you're not hungry at your usual mealtime, delay your meal until you've developed an appetite.

Blood-sugar balance

A steady, even blood-sugar level is key to optimal health, but many people ride the blood-sugar rollercoaster.

Blood-sugar basics

All carbohydrates break down into simple sugars (mainly glucose) in your digestive tract and when they are absorbed into your bloodstream, they increase your blood-sugar levels. How much they rise depends on the type of carbohydrate eaten and how fast it's digested. There are two primary categories of carbohydrate: simple and complex.

Simple carbohydrates (sugar, cereals, refined flour, fruit juice, soft drinks, sweets) have simple structures and are broken down and absorbed quickly, whereas complex carbohydrates (vegetables, legumes, low-sugar whole fruits and wholegrains) have complex structures and contain fibre, so are broken down more slowly.

When you eat simple carbohydrates, your blood-sugar levels rise rapidly and sharply. Although your cells use glucose for energy, it is damaging to your tissues and organs, so your body relies on insulin to move glucose out of your bloodstream and into your cells. The amount of insulin released can be greater than the body needs to bring blood-sugar levels back to a healthy range. This can cause a blood-sugar crash (reactive hypoglycaemia), resulting in symptoms like fatigue, irritability and cravings for sugar or caffeine. A diet high in simple carbohydrates can result in a cycle of highs and lows throughout the day, known colloquially as the blood-sugar rollercoaster.

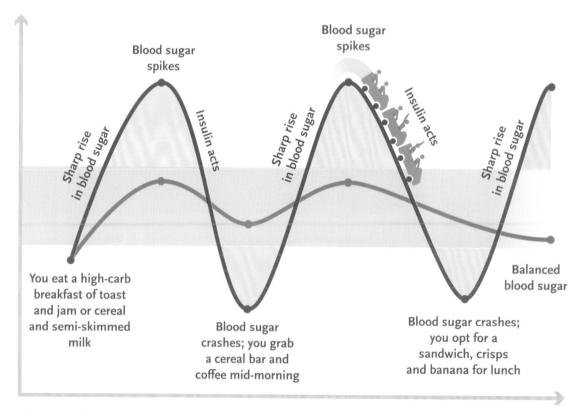

The blood sugar rollercoaster

Insulin resistance

Regularly eating simple carbohydrates forces your body to continuously secrete insulin to regulate blood sugar. Cells are never given a break from insulin's message, and over time their sensitivity decreases, and they stop listening (insulin resistance).

When cells become insulin resistant, blood-sugar regulation becomes more difficult and blood-sugar levels begin to rise. The pancreas works overtime, secreting more and more insulin to normalise blood-sugar levels and eventually, it can no longer keep up. Insulin resistance is the precursor to prediabetes and Type 2 diabetes. It is possible to be insulin resistant without knowing it, as its development begins long before abnormal blood-sugar readings appear on lab tests.

Effect of elevated blood sugar and insulin resistance on fertility

Diets high in sugar and simple carbohydrates correspond with an increased risk of ovulatory infertility. Insulin resistance is associated with poor follicle and egg cell development, implantation failure and poor embryo development. Higher levels of blood sugar and insulin have been linked to lower pregnancy rates during fertility treatment.

Blood-sugar imbalances may also lead to increased production of the stress hormone cortisol, sex hormone imbalances and thyroid dysfunction, which can all affect fertility.

Insulin resistance is a key feature of PCOS. When the ovaries are exposed to high insulin levels in the bloodstream, they begin to alter their hormone production in favour of androgens (male hormones), which disrupts normal ovulation and may lead to irregular cycles and infertility.

Is your blood sugar imbalanced?

Common symptoms of blood-sugar imbalance include:

- Waking a few hours after dropping off, difficult to get back to sleep
- Crave sweets or caffeine
- Binge or uncontrolled eating
- Excessive appetite
- Need coffee or sugar in the afternoon/ to get through the day
- Afternoon tiredness
- Tiredness resolves after eating
- Headaches
- Irritable before meals (hangry!)
- Dizzy or shaky between meals or if meals are delayed
- Excessive thirst and frequent urination (see your doctor)

The blood-sugar solution

One of the most important changes you can make is to significantly reduce or remove sugar and refined foods from your diet. If you've been on the blood-sugar rollercoaster long-term, it may be because you're often tired, stressed, you're not eating enough of the right fuel (complex carbohydrates) or you're eating too much of the wrong fuel (simple carbohydrates), or you might not be eating enough. Removing sugar is challenging and can feel overwhelming, but you can strengthen and support your resolve by keeping your blood sugar balanced:

Eat breakfast to set you up for the day and keep energy steady throughout the morning. Breakfast should be protein-rich and include healthy fat such as avocado, nuts, nut butter or seeds. Include low-sugar whole fruit only as part of your breakfast, in a smoothie or oat bowl, not on its own. Eggs are best (pages 126–130).

Aim for three regular, balanced meals a day. Eating a well-balanced breakfast, lunch and dinner containing high-quality protein, healthy fat and plenty of fibre (vegetables) at every meal helps maintain steady energy levels and keeps you feeling full and satisfied. The Fertility Kitchen plate (pages 72–74) will help with this. Try to avoid snacking – remember constant eating means consistently elevated blood-sugar and insulin levels, which over time can affect hormone balance and ovulation.

Eat nutrient-dense foods and avoid sugar and refined carbohydrates. Whole, real foods pack a lot of nutrition in every serving, help stabilise your blood sugar and nourish your body. Whereas processed foods offer little nutrition or contain 'empty calories', meaning they're high in calories but low in nutrients. These foods are typically addictive, cause blood-sugar spikes and energy dips and won't serve your fertility.

Fibre helps slow digestion and supports blood-sugar balance. Eat at least 30g of fibre every day by including fibre-rich vegetables, nuts, seeds, coconut, legumes and berries. Try making a fibre-rich Seed and nut gluten-free loaf (page 136).

Cinnamon has been shown to have the potential to reduce blood-sugar levels after a meal. It's easy to make cinnamon a feature in your diet. Try a Cinnamon omelette (page 127), Salted almond smoothie (page 138), Cinnamon-chai hot chocolate (page 227) or Almond cinnamon fat bombs (page 215).

Move your body. Both cardio and strength training improve insulin sensitivity and support hormone balance. See pages 111–112 for my movement principles.

Manage stress. Chronic stress can lead to blood-sugar imbalance and insulin resistance. See pages 99–107 for strategies.

Curbing the snack attack

If you find yourself wanting a snack or craving sugar between meals, try the following:

- Review your meal balance. You may need to adjust the balance of protein and healthy fat going forward.
- Drink a glass of water. Hunger can sometimes actually be thirst, which can also cause tiredness and have us reaching for snacks for an energy boost.
- Wait 15 minutes. Hunger can pass, especially if it's actually boredom.
- Move. If time allows, go for a quick walk or do 5 minutes of yoga stretches (pages 104–105). This can be especially helpful if you're feeling tired as exercise gives an energy boost.
- Eat. If you are genuinely hungry, then eat a well-balanced snack, such as:
  1–2 fat bombs of your choice (page 215)
  1 tablespoon nut butter and a green apple
  60g (½ cup) mixed nuts or homemade Granola (pages 140–141)
  ½ jar (100g) wild salmon in olive oil
  Handful of olives
  1 carrot cut into sticks with 1–2 tablespoons Hummus (pages 200–201)
  1–2 hard-boiled egg(s)

If nothing but sweetness will do, try 1–2 squares of 90% cocoa solids dark chocolate dipped into almond butter or tahini. This is a client favourite! Or, if you're a lover of gummy sweets, then try 1–2 Gut-lovin' gummies (pages 222–223), which include minimal sweetness.

Understand food labels

Familiarise yourself with the words that mean sugar on food labels (there are over 70! See the Appendix on page 232). It is recommended you consume a maximum of 7 teaspoons of sugar per day. But how can you tell how much sugar is in the foods you buy? Here's a quick example of a granola label:

Nutrition	Per 40g serving	Per 100g
Energy kJ	772	1930
Energy kcal	184	460
Fat	7.2	18
of which saturates	0.8	2.1
Carbohydrates	24.4	61
of which sugars	4.8	12

Calculate the percentage of sugar

Look at the 'Per 100g' column on a nutrition label, then find the carbohydrates row and underneath you'll see 'of which are sugars'. This equates to the percentage of sugar in the food. You can see in the above example the food contains 12% sugar. As a general guideline, choose foods with less than 5g of sugar per 100g (5% sugar or less). This will remove most processed foods from your shopping trolley.

Calculate the sugar content in teaspoons

Move to the 'Per serving' column and again look for carbohydrates, of which are sugars. 4.2g sugar = 1 teaspoon, so divide the sugar content by 4.2 to get the number of teaspoons per serving. But you will need to account for larger than suggested serving sizes, so in this example, the serving size is 40g. However, people typically serve themselves double this, so the number of teaspoons in this example will be 9.6 (4.8 x 2) divided by 4.2, which is just over 2 teaspoons. Then you'll need to account for toppings (fruit, yoghurt, perhaps a little honey), so you can see how easy it is to consume your daily recommended sugar intake in a single meal, especially if you are eating commercial breakfast cereals and adding things like dried fruit and sweeteners.

Liver detoxification

Many organs are involved in detoxification, including your liver, lungs, kidneys, skin and gut, but it is your liver that undertakes by far the greatest share of the work. As well as transforming the natural waste products of metabolism and the toxins you encounter daily, it also processes the hormones your body no longer needs. Efficient detoxification plays a central role in hormonal balance, the menstrual cycle and fertility.

Detoxification basics

Toxins can be created internally (natural waste products of metabolism and hormones like oestrogen), or you can be exposed to them in the environment (pollution, cigarette smoke, plastics, pesticides, household chemicals and personal-care products). How much these toxins affect your health depends not only on your level of exposure, but also on how well your detoxification system is functioning.

Detoxification is a two-phase process that enables toxins to be safely excreted from your body. During phase 1, highly reactive molecules (free radicals) are produced and they can be potentially more harmful to your body than the toxin was to start with. They create oxidative stress and can damage your cells. Your body requires an abundance of antioxidants to help protect your liver and the rest of your body from damage caused by these molecules. Egg and sperm cells are particularly sensitive to oxidative stress and require a high volume of antioxidants to support their development. If your liver is dealing with a high level of toxins or there are not enough resources (nutrients) to properly process them, all resources will be preferentially used for liver detoxification, rather than for other (less important) functions such as reproduction.

In phase 2, the molecules produced in phase 1 are prepared for excretion and this requires dietary amino acids (protein). A nutrient-rich diet is crucial for optimal detoxification, as well as high-quality protein, detoxification pathways require an array of micronutrients, especially the B vitamins (particularly vitamins B6, B9 (folate) and B12), antioxidants, choline, iron and magnesium.

Oestrogen metabolism

Your body removes oestrogen from your body via phase 1 and phase 2 detoxification and eliminates it through your gut. This requires optimal gut health and a healthy microbiome. Healthy gut bacteria assist with the safe removal of oestrogen via your stool, whereas unhealthy bacteria can obstruct oestrogen metabolism by making an enzyme called beta-glucuronidase, which reactivates oestrogen, allowing it to be reabsorbed. Similarly, if you are constipated your body won't be able to excrete it as intended.

This can lead to recirculation of oestrogen, resulting in hormonal imbalance with symptoms like heavy periods, PMS and cyclical breast tenderness.

Endometriosis and fibroids are oestrogen-dependent conditions and hormonal imbalances sit at the heart of PCOS, so liver detoxification support is key if you have one of these conditions.

The bathtub analogy

Think of your body as a bathtub and everything that enters your body is represented by the water from the tap, and everything that leaves your body is represented by the water draining away. Your body can handle a certain amount of toxins coming in (the water), because it is simultaneously getting rid of toxins (via the drain). If too much water is coming in and not enough draining away, what might happen? Overflow! To ensure your bathtub doesn't overflow, you can decrease the flow in (toxins you ingest and encounter) and increase the flow out (by supporting detoxification).

Is your liver demanding your attention?

These symptoms suggest that your liver may benefit from detoxification support:

- Headaches
- Night sweats
- Fatigue and sluggishness
- Acne and skin eruptions
- Low mood and irritability
- Sensitivity to chemicals, odours or pollution
- Bloating, wind and constipation
- Gallbladder removal or gallbladder issues

Symptoms of elevated oestrogen
- Heavy or painful periods
- PMS
- Mood swings
- Feeling emotional or crying for no reason,

especially one week before your period

- Weight gain around your hips, bum and thighs
- Bloating, especially around ovulation and during the second half of your cycle
- Constipation, especially before your period
- Fibroids or endometriosis

Optimising liver function

Supporting detoxification is an easy way to start feeling better fast. Try the following simple suggestions for improved mood, energy, skin and periods:

Optimise your gut health. Avoid constipation – remember, you need to open your bowels every day to prevent reabsorption of toxins. Addressing leaky gut

Smart supplements for optimal liver function

Under the guidance of a nutritional therapist, consider the following supplements to help support your liver:

- B-VITAMINS are needed to support detoxification pathways. MTHFR is a gene that produces an enzyme necessary for the metabolism of folate and vitamin B12, for methylation, detoxification and protection from oxidative stress damage to cells and DNA. Variations in this gene are common; it is estimated that up to 60 per cent of people have a reduced ability to use folic acid (synthetic folate) due to their genetics and therefore require the active form, L-methylfolate. Look for a methylated B-complex supplement or check that your prenatal multivitamin contains active B vitamins and not folic acid (see pages 80–81 for my recommendation).
- BROCCOLI SEED EXTRACT has been shown to support liver function by reducing oxidative stress. It is rich in

sulforaphane, which supports oestrogen metabolism.

- LIPOSOMAL GLUTATHIONE is a well-absorbed form of glutathione – your body's master antioxidant. Your liver requires significant amounts to perform detoxification. You can get a small amount from food such as spinach, avocado and asparagus, but a supplement is the best way to increase glutathione within your body.
- MAGNESIUM (CITRATE) before bed if you are constipated to help support healthy bowel movements.
- MILK THISTLE. Silymarin is a compound in milk thistle that may support liver health and protect against liver damage due to its antioxidant and anti-inflammatory properties.
- N-ACETYL CYSTEINE (NAC) is needed to make and replenish glutathione and plays an important role in your body's detoxification processes. It may also help improve fertility in men, and in women with PCOS.

and supporting microbial diversity is also key (see Start with your gut on pages 13–21).

Eat cruciferous vegetables (broccoli, Brussels sprouts, cabbage, cauliflower, collard greens, kale, rocket and watercress). These vegetables contain the plant nutrients indole-3-carbinol (I3C) and sulforaphane, which support both phases of detoxification. Broccoli sprouts (see Pantry staples on page 83) are especially high in sulforaphane and can be sprinkled on soups, burgers, salads and curry. Aim to include 30–50g (1 cup) of cruciferous vegetables with each meal.

Eat the rainbow to support your liver with a wide range of antioxidants and plant nutrients (use the tracker on pages 52–53). Focus on leafy greens, berries, beetroot, citrus zest, ginger, onions and garlic. Use herbs and spices in cooking, especially turmeric (for curcumin), coriander, rosemary and parsley.

Increase dietary fibre. Eating adequate fibre (a minimum of 30g daily) and staying hydrated supports regular bowel movements and oestrogen excretion and provides food for your gut bacteria, helping to support bacterial diversity and crowd out the gut bacteria that make beta-glucuronidase. Try my fibre-rich Seed and nut gluten-free loaf (page 136) and eat plenty of vegetables (see veggie recipes on pages 184–199).

Eat high-quality protein with every meal. Your liver needs protein for the amino acids that power its detoxification pathways. Include organic grass-fed meats and pasture-raised eggs, wild-caught fish, organic legumes, nuts and seeds (these are especially important if you don't eat meat). Use The Fertility Kitchen plate (pages 72–74) to help build your meals.

Eat monounsaturated fats and polyunsaturated fats from olive oil, avocados, oily fish, nuts and seeds as your primary fat source. These fats support bile production, which helps excrete toxins in phase 2 detoxification. Include 1–2 tablespoons with each meal and 1 portion of oily fish as your protein source two to three times a week.

Drink dandelion root tea, which is thought to promote bile flow and support liver function. Enjoy 1–3 cups daily.

Check for iron deficiency, especially if you have heavy periods. Iron is a key component of detoxification enzymes. Haem iron from red meat, liver, darker poultry meat, oily fish and eggs is the most readily absorbed. Absorption of non-haem iron from dark-green leafy vegetables is

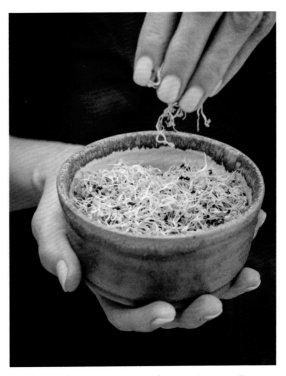

Use broccoli sprouts to garnish soup (page 146), as a burger topping (pages 177–178) or sprinkle on salad.

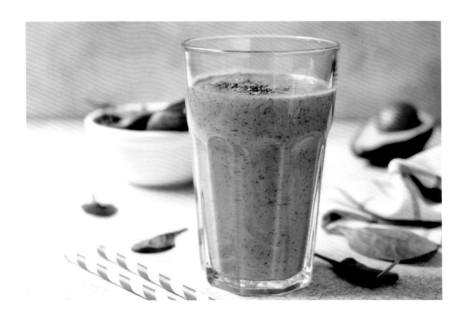

Show your liver some love with The fresh green smoothie (page 138).

improved with vitamin C-rich foods such as berries, bell peppers, kiwi and broccoli. Test your ferritin (iron storage protein) level via your GP or online blood-testing service (see Resources on page 235).

Minimise alcohol as it raises oestrogen levels and rapidly depletes glutathione (your master antioxidant) in the liver. If you want to have a drink, stick to an occasional small glass (125ml) of good-quality organic red wine with dinner (for more guidance on alcohol, see page 71).

Avoid inflammatory and trans fats, including vegetable oils and hydrogenated vegetable oils, found in margarine and other butter substitutes, processed snack foods, frozen dinners and fast food.

Avoid processed foods, which may contain chemical additives such as colourings, sweeteners, flavour enhancers and high amounts of salt.

Minimise or avoid sugar. Sugar increases inflammation and burdens the liver. See Blood-sugar balance on pages 22–26 for strategies for help with this.

Move your body. Exercise improves circulation and helps move your lymph. You also eliminate toxins through your skin in your sweat. See pages 111–112 for more on exercise.

Castor oil packs enhance liver function, stimulate the healthy flow of lymph, and support detoxification pathways (see Resources on page 233). Make your own by saturating a flannel with castor oil, fold it in three and place it across your abdomen with a towel and hot water bottle on top. A castor oil pack is the perfect time to practise meditation, breathing techniques or legs up the wall yoga pose (page 104) for deep relaxation. Note: castor oil packs are not suitable in pregnancy so stop these when you get a positive pregnancy test. It is also not advisable to use castor oil packs during your period.

Epsom salts bath. Add 1–2 cups of salts to a warm bath with 3–5 drops of organic lavender essential oil and relax for 30 minutes. Enjoy two to three times a week. Meditate at the same time for deep relaxation.

Dry body brushing helps stimulate the movement of lymph fluid and encourages detoxification from the largest organ of your body – your skin. Use a natural-bristle brush and start with your feet and work your way up, using upward strokes moving towards your heart. The best time to brush is before a shower or bath in the morning.

Minimise your exposure to toxins from pesticides, plastics, household cleaners, cosmetics and body products (pages 112–116).

Thyroid function

Your thyroid gland, along with your reproductive glands, is part of the endocrine system. These glands secrete hormones that affect various body parts and organs. Your thyroid is the master gland of metabolism. It uses dietary iodine and the amino acid tyrosine to produce thyroid hormones (inactive T4 and active T3) that deliver oxygen and energy to every cell in your body. T4 must be converted to T3 to become active in your body.

Your thyroid operates in a feedback loop with the hypothalamus and pituitary gland in your brain. It is comparable to the thermostat in your house, causing the heat to go on or off to maintain a set temperature. When low thyroid hormone levels are detected, the hypothalamus stimulates the pituitary to release thyroid-stimulating hormone (TSH) and prolactin. TSH signals to your thyroid gland to make more thyroid hormone. When increasing blood levels of thyroid hormones are detected, TSH production drops and production of thyroid hormones slows.

Understanding thyroid dysfunction

Hypothyroidism (underactive thyroid) means there is too little thyroid hormone. The most common cause is an autoimmune condition called Hashimoto's disease, where the immune system mistakenly targets the thyroid gland and makes thyroid antibodies that cause inflammation (thyroiditis) and gradually destroy it. The gland becomes incapable of producing enough thyroid hormone, resulting in hypothyroidism. It is not known what causes Hashimoto's, however, gluten sensitivity or coeliac disease, environmental toxins, stress and nutritional deficiencies may be contributing factors.

Other causes of hypothyroidism include surgical removal of the thyroid, congenital hypothyroidism (absent or underdeveloped at birth), medication, thyroiditis (inflammation), infection (such as Epstein Barr), iodine deficiency and exposure to environmental toxins such as fluoride or perchlorate (found in non-stick cookware).

Hyperthyroidism (overactive thyroid) means the thyroid is producing an excess of thyroid hormone. The most common cause is an autoimmune condition called Grave's disease, which is associated with the development of a goitre (enlarged thyroid gland). In Grave's, antibodies bind to the thyroid gland resulting in overproduction of thyroid hormone.

Some people with Hashimoto's experience phases of hyperthyroidism, known as Hashitoxicosis, caused by the destruction of the thyroid gland. Other causes of hyperthyroidism include medication (e.g. over-dosage of thyroid hormone replacement medication) and supplements containing thyroid hormone. Most thyroid conditions, or the treatments for them, result in hypothyroidism, and this is a common primary contributing factor to fertility issues.

The thyroid-fertility connection

Normal thyroid function is essential to your ability to conceive and sustain a healthy pregnancy. An undiagnosed or poorly managed thyroid condition can affect fertility in various ways, resulting in anovulatory cycles (lack of ovulation), luteal phase defect (short luteal phase and insufficient progesterone), high prolactin levels (hyperprolactinemia) and sex hormone imbalances. Hyperprolactinemia can interfere with normal production of other hormones, such as oestrogen and progesterone, and affect fertility by preventing ovulation and causing irregular or missed periods.

Hypothyroidism is associated with decreased levels of sex hormone binding globulin (SHBG). SHBG binds to oestrogen, and low levels can result in elevated oestrogen, which can increase the need for thyroid hormone at the cellular level (even when circulating blood levels appear normal), because oestrogen competes with thyroid hormones to attach to thyroid receptor sites throughout the body. Elevated oestrogen can therefore block the transportation of thyroid hormone into cells.

The prevalence of Hashimoto's is significantly higher amongst infertile women than amongst fertile women, especially those with endometriosis, ovarian dysfunction and unexplained infertility. Thyroid autoimmunity is associated with recurrent miscarriage; the presence of thyroid antibodies doubles the risk of recurrent miscarriage in women with otherwise normal thyroid function.

During pregnancy, your thyroid must expand its function to encompass the needs of both you and your developing baby. This continues throughout pregnancy but is especially important during the first trimester as foetal brain development relies on thyroid hormone, but the foetus doesn't produce its own until around 12 weeks' gestation.

How do you know if your thyroid needs support?

Symptoms reflect the lack of oxygen and energy that results from too little thyroid hormone:

- Fatigue
- Feeling cold, cold hands and feet
- Sluggish digestion or constipation
- Hair loss
- Loss of the outer edge of your eyebrows
- Weight gain
- Swelling and puffiness
- Brain fog
- Poor memory
- Slow pulse
- Low blood pressure

Menstrual symptoms

- Long or irregular cycles
- Anovulatory cycles (lack of ovulation)
- Heavy or prolonged bleeding
- Irregular bleeding
- Luteal phase defect

Associated conditions

- Elevated prolactin
- Unexplained infertility
- Endometriosis
- PCOS
- Recurrent miscarriage
- Family history of thyroid disease or autoimmune conditions
- Existing autoimmune conditions (e.g. coeliac disease)

Understanding thyroid testing

Understanding thyroid testing will help you advocate for yourself. Seventy per cent of women with hypothyroidism have no symptoms. The most common thyroid blood test measures the amount of TSH in your blood. Values are interpreted using a reference or 'normal' range. The reference range typically runs from 0.5 mIU/L to 4.5 mIU/L. TSH above normal suggests hypothyroidism, while TSH below normal suggests hyperthyroidism. However, an optimal TSH for fertility and pregnancy is thought to be ≤2.5 mIU/L.

Other tests can also be used to assess thyroid health, such as thyroid hormones (T4 and T3) and the presence of thyroid antibodies. Elevated thyroid peroxidase antibodies (TPOAb) suggest inflammation of the thyroid gland and are thought to be detectable in approximately 95 per cent of people with Hashimoto's. Some people have elevated TPOAb with normal TSH and T4/T3, so it is important to test antibodies to rule out autoimmunity, especially if you experience any of the associated conditions mentioned above. You may be able to arrange comprehensive thyroid testing via your GP or if not, you can use an online blood testing service (see Resources on page 235). Seek the support of a nutritional therapist if you need help interpreting results.

Optimising thyroid function

Optimise liver function. Your liver is the major site of thyroid hormone conversion (inactive T4 to active T3) – about 60 per cent of the conversion happens here. Supporting liver detoxification can be helpful in facilitating this process and alleviating symptoms of low thyroid function. See page 26 for liver support.

Optimise gut health. About 20 per cent of thyroid hormone conversion occurs in the gut, so it's essential to make sure that your gut is functioning well. It is especially important to support your gut health and calm inflammation if there is an autoimmune component (elevated antibodies). See pages 13–21 for gut support.

Eat a nutrient-rich diet. Certain minerals are required for healthy thyroid function, including iodine, iron, magnesium, selenium and zinc. Eat the rainbow for the wide array of nutrients needed for optimal thyroid health. Regular high-quality protein is also essential for the amino acid tyrosine needed to make thyroid hormones. Use The Fertility Kitchen plate (pages 72–74) and Eat a rainbow tracker (pages 52–53) to increase nutrient density and diversity.

Support blood-sugar balance (pages 22–24) as thyroid hormones play an important role in blood-sugar balance, and hypothyroidism can alter glucose metabolism.

Include dietary iodine. I generally don't recommend an iodine supplement beyond what is included in a prenatal multivitamin (check that yours does include it as many don't), as iodine may cause a flare of the autoimmune response in those with Hashimoto's. Instead, I recommend being diligent about including iodine-rich foods in your diet to meet your iodine needs. Dulse seaweed flakes are a good source and can be sprinkled onto soups, salads, fish or stir-fries (see Pantry staples on page 87). Include 2 teaspoons a day for a small amount of dietary iodine. Fish is another good source (see pages 161–164 for fish recipes), it is also a reliable source of zinc, which is needed for healthy thyroid function.

Include iron-rich foods. Iron is crucial for the synthesis of T4. The most bio-available iron is haem iron from red meat, especially liver (try my hidden recipes on pages 168 and 178. Liver also contains vitamin A, a co-factor in thyroid function), the darker meat from poultry, oily fish and eggs. Sources of vegetarian iron include dark-green leafy vegetables and legumes. It is better absorbed with vitamin C, so include vitamin C-rich foods (berries, bell peppers, citrus, kiwi) at the same time. Don't supplement without checking ferritin levels first. Ferritin is your iron storage protein, the reference range is 15–150 ug/L, but an optimal level is 45–85 ug/L. Arrange

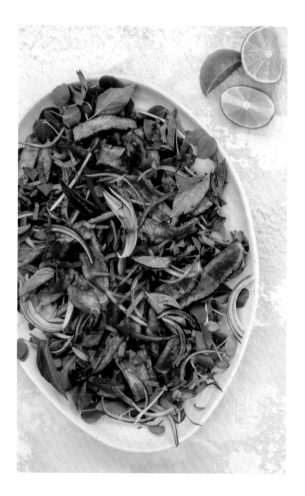

This Thai beef salad (page 157) is crammed with iron.

testing via your GP or an online blood-testing service (see Resources on page 235).

Avoid gluten. Individuals with thyroid autoimmunity have an almost fivefold increased risk of developing coeliac disease, and this can happen at any time. Gluten protein and thyroid tissue have similar amino acid (protein) sequences, so this is a way that your body can get confused. If you start producing antibodies to gluten, you can also start producing antibodies to thyroid tissue in a process known as molecular mimicry. To help you avoid gluten I have included a handy list of swaps (see page 17). Plus, all the recipes in this book are gluten-free.

Avoid soy. Soy contains goitrogens, which block the uptake of iodine in the thyroid. Find swaps on page 19.

Avoid raw cruciferous vegetables, which also contain goitrogens. Cooking bypasses this issue, so don't avoid them completely.

Detox your environment. Toxins such as perchlorate, chlorine and fluoride may be specifically problematic for thyroid health. Evidence associates the chemicals used in non-stick cookware (perfluorinated compounds) with sub-optimal thyroid function. Filtering your drinking water and removing non-stick cookware (pages 114–115) are a high priority if you have thyroid dysfunction.

Manage stress to enhance hormonal balance. The thyroid and adrenals are connected through the hypothalamic-pituitary-adrenal (HPA) axis and the hypothalamus-pituitary-thyroid (HPT) axis. An excessive output of the adrenal hormone cortisol (due to chronic stress) may therefore contribute to low thyroid function. Think of the endocrine system as an orchestra: when parts of it are out of tune, the rest go out of sync. As the conductor, it is your job to make sure your hormonal system is working harmoniously. Stress is a factor that can tip the balance. See pages 99–106 for strategies to help manage this.

Move your body to promote thyroid function and thyroid hormone sensitivity and support production of SHBG. See pages 111–112 for movement support.

Smart supplements for thyroid health

Under the guidance of a nutritional therapist, consider these supplements:

- PRENATAL MULTIVITAMIN to help address any nutritional deficiencies and build nutrient stores (selenium, zinc and iodine are particularly important for thyroid health, so check that your prenatal multivitamin contains these nutrients). See pages 80–81 for my recommendation.
- SELENIUM if you have elevated thyroid antibodies. Selenium protects the thyroid from inflammation and oxidative stress that suppresses function and damages thyroid tissue.
- VITAMIN D deficiency may contribute to the development of autoimmune thyroid conditions.
  Check your levels via your GP or online blood-testing service (see Resources on page 235) and supplement if necessary (pages 80–81).

Egg quality

Egg quality is a common concern when trying to conceive. Many women come to see me after they've had their anti-mullerian hormone (AMH) tested and are panicking about the results. AMH is a marker for ovarian reserve and a low level suggests low egg count, or diminished ovarian reserve (DOR), but it doesn't tell the whole story. It's important to know this, especially if you've been told you have low fertility based solely on your AMH.

Think of your egg reserve as a basket of eggs. You're typically born with a full basket and they get used up over your lifetime. If you have DOR, your basket is starting to empty. However, although low AMH suggests DOR, it's not definite and it doesn't tell you anything about the quality of the eggs in your basket. Therefore, AMH doesn't accurately predict natural fertility, it just gives an indication of whether you have the expected number of eggs in your basket for your age. Age remains the best measure of egg quality because both quantity and quality decline with age.

Egg quality refers to the capability of an egg to be fertilised and go through the developmental stages to form a viable embryo. This is largely determined by two factors: chromosomes and the energy supply of the egg. Your egg cells exist in a 'resting' state for most of your life. The process of follicle growth starts with the recruitment of primordial follicles into a 'growing pool' around one year before ovulation. Approximately three months before ovulation, follicular growth and development accelerate. A dominant follicle is selected at around 15–20 days prior to ovulation. These months before ovulation

(at least three, ideally one year) represent a window of opportunity where you can influence your egg quality by optimising the environment in which your follicles grow and develop.

Factors that influence egg quality

Low androgens. Androgens (male sex hormones) such as testosterone play a key role in the maturation of ovarian follicles. Androgens naturally decline with age. For example, testosterone declines by 50 per cent in women between the ages of 20 and 40. Low androgen levels have been associated with poor follicular growth, DOR and primary ovarian insufficiency (POI).

Dehydroepiandrosterone (DHEA) is a primary adrenal hormone that converts into androgen hormones, so it plays an important role in follicular development as a precursor hormone. DHEA levels naturally decline with age. Other factors that may reduce DHEA include stress, medications and autoimmunity.

Symptoms of low androgens

These symptoms are associated with low testosterone:

- **Low libido**
- **Difficulty reaching orgasm**
- **Fatigue and lack of motivation (no 'get-up-and-go')**
- **Depression or mood swings**
- **Loss of muscle tone or trouble gaining muscle**

Oxidative stress and telomere shortening

Oxidative stress is caused by an imbalance between the production and accumulation of reactive oxygen species (ROS), also known as free radicals, in your cells and tissues and the ability of your body to detoxify them. Free radicals are unstable molecules that can harm your cells and have been shown to affect egg cell maturation and fertilisation, embryo development and pregnancy, and it is thought that oxidative stress plays a role in the age-related decline in fertility. Free radicals damage cells and deplete ATP – energy vital to egg development and embryo viability.

Oxidative stress has been associated with endometriosis, PCOS and unexplained infertility. Pregnancy complications such as miscarriage, recurrent pregnancy loss and preeclampsia may also develop in response to oxidative stress.

Telomeres are found at the ends of chromosomes and protect DNA from damage. Telomere shortening is thought to influence female fertility, affecting both egg quantity and quality as we age. Studies have linked short telomere length with IVF failure, embryo fragmentation, chromosome abnormalities, DOR and recurrent pregnancy loss.

Oxidative stress plays a key role in telomere shortening, and egg cells are particularly vulnerable due to the prolonged interval between their development and ovulation. A poor lifestyle can affect telomere length: smoking, environmental toxins, sedentary lifestyle, obesity, stress and poor diet all increase oxidative stress and telomere shortening.

Symptoms of oxidative stress

These symptoms are associated with the ageing process:

- Unexplained tiredness
- Brain fog or poor memory
- Frequent headaches and susceptibility to noise
- Inflammatory conditions
- Decreased eyesight
- Wrinkles and grey hair

Impaired mitochondrial function

Mitochondria are your cells' powerhouses; they produce about 90 per cent of the energy that cells need to survive. Each egg cell contains over 100,000 mitochondria (whereas sperm cells only have a few hundred) because significant energy is required for rapid cell division in the embryo. Egg cells in older women show accumulations of mitochondrial DNA mutations that impair function and aren't compatible with normal, healthy fertility.

After fertilisation, the embryo grows rapidly by cell division. The cells divide, but the mitochondria do not. Instead, the initial number is split with each division so that a few weeks after conception each cell has roughly 200 mitochondria. This can expose defective mitochondria, which will be removed. When this occurs in just one or two cells it's unlikely to cause an issue, however, when enough mitochondria are defective in enough cells, the pregnancy won't be viable.

Coenzyme Q10 is the primary antioxidant your cells make to protect and support mitochondria. In order to produce it, cells need an amino acid called tyrosine, several vitamins and trace minerals. A deficiency in any of these impairs your cells' ability to produce Coenzyme Q10.

Coenzyme Q10 deficiency is thought to contribute to age-related infertility, because production naturally declines with age (as early as your thirties). Deficiency reduces energy production in egg cells, so when

Smart supplements for egg quality

Under the guidance of a nutritional therapist, consider the following supplements:

- **ALPHA LIPOIC ACID** is a powerful antioxidant shown to improve mitochondrial function and has beneficial effects on egg quality, fertilisation and embryo development.
- **COENZYME Q10** supports mitochondrial function in egg cells. Although you get a small amount of Coenzyme Q10 from food, it isn't enough, so supplements become important, especially with age. Ubiquinol is the reduced form of Coenzyme Q10 and is thought to be better absorbed.
- **DHEA** supplementation is an option for some women, although this needs to be arranged through a fertility clinic as hormones are prescription-only in the UK. DHEA can support testosterone production, so women frequently benefit from taking this when their levels are low, and it may improve egg quality.
- **GLUTATHIONE** is a powerful antioxidant made by your body's cells that helps shield eggs from the damage caused by oxidative stress during follicular development, so egg quality is dependent on it. Glutathione levels decrease as a result of ageing, stress and toxin exposure. Supplemental glutathione may support egg quality by reducing oxidative stress.

- **N-ACETYL CYSTEINE (NAC)** is important for replenishing glutathione, your body's master antioxidant, supports mitochondrial function and may be helpful for women with PCOS.
- **PRENATAL MULTIVITAMIN.** A high-quality prenatal multivitamin will contain methylated B vitamins, such as folate, vitamin B12 and vitamin B6, as well as antioxidant nutrients such as vitamin C, vitamin E, selenium and zinc, which help protect egg cells from oxidative stress. See pages 80–81 for my recommendation.
- **MYO-INOSITOL** may help support egg quality and promote ovarian function in women with PCOS. It may also be helpful for irregular ovulation, recurrent miscarriage or issues with egg maturity during IVF.
- **PYRROLOQUINOLINE QUINONE (PQQ)** is thought to promote mitochondrial function and the cellular development of new mitochondria and therefore support cellular energy production and in turn, egg quality.

fertilised, conditions are sub-optimal for embryo development. If there is sufficient cellular energy to stay above the threshold for miscarriage, the embryo will continue developing. However, in some embryos that escape miscarriage, cellular energy can be insufficient to properly separate the chromosomes during cell division. An example of this is trisomy 21 (Down syndrome), where there are three copies of chromosome 21, which is more common in older women.

Optimising egg quality

These recommendations are focused on supporting androgens (to help promote the growth of very early-stage follicles), reducing oxidative stress and optimising mitochondrial health.

Optimise liver detoxification and gut health to promote elimination of toxins and manage inflammation (pages 26–31).

Manage blood sugar to avoid blood-sugar and insulin spikes, and manage inflammation (pages 22–26). Use The

Fertility Kitchen plate (pages 72–74) to build your meals and ensure that you are eating an appropriate balance of carbohydrate, protein and fat to support follicular development.

Eat an abundance of antioxidant nutrients. Antioxidants are molecules that fight free radicals in your body. Your body makes its own antioxidants, but they are also found in food, especially fruit and vegetables. Make plants the foundation of your plate and eat as many colours as possible. Include herbs and spices, which provide concentrated nutrition. Use The Fertility Kitchen plate (pages 72–74) and Eat a rainbow tracker (pages 52–53).

Focus on monounsaturated fats, especially olive oil for oleic acid, which is found in developing egg cells.

Eat oily fish two to three times a week for omega-3 fats. Read more on pages 62–63.

Include orange-coloured vegetables and fruits such as carrots, orange peppers, pumpkin, sweet potatoes, turmeric, apricots, blood oranges, cantaloupe,

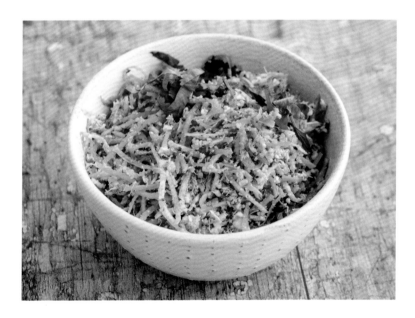

This Veggie rice (page 197) will help up your intake of those all-important carotenes.

mandarins, passion fruit and papaya. These contain carotenoid compounds, antioxidants that are particularly concentrated in the ovaries. One study found the presence of up to fourteen different carotenoids in ovarian tissue.

Maca is thought to support healthy testosterone (and oestrogen) levels. Maca can be taken as a supplement, or you can add maca powder to smoothies, oat bowls, energy bars and more. I use maca powder in the Salted cashew and maca oats (page 133), Cinnamon omelettes (page 127) and Adaptogenic cinnamon-chai hot chocolate (page 227).

Aromatase inhibitors may protect testosterone by blocking aromatase enzymes. Aromatase enzymes convert testosterone into oestrogen; this may happen too efficiently and deplete testosterone. Aromatase inhibitors can be found in foods such as button mushrooms, cruciferous vegetables (broccoli, Brussels sprouts, cabbage, collard greens, kale, rocket and watercress) and green tea extract – try a Revitalising matcha latte (page 225).

Avoid foods that increase free radicals. These include polycyclic aromatic hydrocarbons (PAHs) from burned and barbecued food; nitrosamines found in processed meats, such as bacon; acrylamides, which can form during high-temperature cooking such as frying; and oxidised and trans fats found in vegetable oils, margarine, shortening and anything made with these, such as processed foods.

Manage stress. Ninety per cent of your DHEA is made by your adrenal glands.

Chronic stress can affect DHEA and, in turn, your androgens. If stress is a factor for you, then you may need to support your adrenals to support androgens. See pages 100–107 for strategies to manage stress.

Optimise sleep. See pages 107–110 for supportive strategies if sleep is an issue for you.

Exercise, especially strength training, helps build muscle and support testosterone production. Moderate exercise has been shown to decrease oxidative stress and improve mitochondrial function, whereas strenuous exercise increases oxidative stress. See pages 111–112 for my movement principles.

Minimise exposure to toxins from pollution, household and personal care products (pages 112–116).

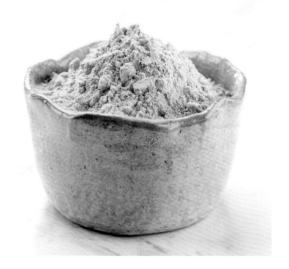

Add maca powder to hot drinks, smoothies, oats and bakes.

It takes two

Men provide half the genetic material needed to conceive and grow a healthy baby, so it's just as important for men to prepare for conception as it is for women. A man's diet and lifestyle can profoundly impact his ability to conceive. Sperm is in constant production in a process called spermatogenesis, which takes around 74 days. This represents a window of opportunity in which to focus on supporting sperm quality to maximise fertility potential.

How male fertility is typically evaluated

Men should be offered a physical examination to assess for anatomical abnormalities such as varicocele. A varicocele is an enlargement of veins in the scrotum, like a varicose vein in the leg. It's a common cause of male infertility and may result in reduced motility, abnormal form and, over time, reduced sperm concentration. In my experience, men are rarely offered a physical examination; request this if not offered as the prevalence of varicocele in infertile men may be as high as 40 per cent.

Semen analysis remains the primary investigation of male fertility and uses three parameters to assess sperm function:

- **Sperm count** (number of sperm present in 1ml semen) – at least 15 million per ml is considered normal.
- **Motility** (ability of the sperm to move efficiently) – typically at least 50 per cent will demonstrate normal motility.
- **Morphology** (percentage with a normal size and shape) – normal semen should contain a minimum of 4 per cent sperm with expected form.

However, there is controversy over what constitutes 'normal' parameters, and although semen analysis provides useful information, it doesn't provide insight into the functional potential of the sperm to fertilise an egg. While the results may correlate with fertility, a semen analysis is not a direct measure of fertility.

The standards for normal values in semen analysis do not reflect average values but are instead determined using the bottom 5 per cent as a cut-off point. This means it is the minimum standard for pregnancy. In one study, 15 per cent of men with male infertility were found to have normal semen analysis results, which shows the limitations of semen analysis.

One of the main factors affecting male fertility is DNA fragmentation in sperm. This is the separation or breakdown of DNA strands within the sperm. It's very important to consider the effects of sperm DNA damage, since half of your future baby's genetics come from the father. DNA damage can have adverse effects on fertilisation and embryo development, is associated with failure to conceive, longer time to pregnancy, poor outcome following intrauterine insemination (IUI), miscarriage and pregnancy loss after IVF and ICSI. It has been established that if sperm DNA fragmentation exceeds 30 per cent, sperm quality is significantly reduced.

It can also be useful to test LH, FSH, testosterone and prolactin, especially if sperm count is low, as these hormones are responsible for spermatogenesis.

Factors that influence sperm quality

Oxidative stress. Like egg cells, sperm are susceptible to oxidative stress during the 2–3 months of their development and maturation. Oxidation is what happens to a sliced apple when it turns brown and to the human body as it degenerates. It occurs continuously within the body, particularly during cell metabolism within the mitochondria. Sperm are especially vulnerable, as to be motile, they need to have very high metabolisms, exposing them to significant free-radical damage in their short life spans.

A healthy body can manage a certain level of oxidative stress as it can make antioxidant compounds and use antioxidants from food, if dietary intake is sufficient. Sometimes, the balance of free radicals and antioxidants is imbalanced, leading to excessive oxidative stress, which can influence sperm quality and damage sperm DNA.

A variety of factors may contribute to oxidative stress; these include lifestyle factors such as smoking, recreational drugs, alcohol intake, obesity, testicular heat stress, psychological stress, age, diet and caffeine intake.

Smoking. We all know by now that smoking isn't good for health, which means it's not good for fertility either. Cigarette smoking is an established potential risk factor for reduced male fertility. Cigarettes contain free radicals at levels that can overwhelm the body's natural antioxidant defences. Increased levels of free radicals in semen expose sperm to oxidative stress, which can impair function and compromise male fertility. Smoking is associated with DNA damage, chromosome abnormalities and mutations in sperm.

Recreational drugs such as marijuana, cocaine, anabolic-androgenic steroids, opiates and methamphetamines have been shown to have adverse effects on male fertility and are linked to decreased sperm concentration, count and motility, and abnormal morphology.

Alcohol intake. Sorry guys, but alcohol intake has also been associated with reduced male fertility. Research links alcohol intake with lower semen volume and increased abnormal forms. Alcohol appears to interfere with the production of the hormones involved in spermatogenesis (FSH, LH and testosterone), affecting sperm production, morphology and maturation. However, the negative effects seem to be dependent on the intake amount, as studies have shown a correlation between a drop in spermatogenesis and increased levels of alcohol intake. Alcohol consumption has been found to be higher in men with very low sperm count and no sperm, compared to fertile controls.

Overweight and obesity are associated with low sperm count, low motility, DNA fragmentation and abnormal morphology and put men at a greater risk of infertility. Excess body fat may disrupt hormonal balance, resulting in impaired spermatogenesis. Increased scrotal fat has been associated with oxidative stress due to testicular heat stress, which may impair spermatogenesis and cause DNA damage.

Testicular heat stress. There is a reason the testicles hang outside the body. Our body temperature is 37°C, but spermatogenesis is most efficient at 34°C. Elevated scrotal temperature may impair sperm production and cause oxidative stress and DNA damage. Prolonged hours of sitting, intense cycling, exposure to radiation, varicocele and undescended testicles can all result in testicular heat stress. Exposure to radiofrequency electromagnetic fields (RF-EMF) from mobile phones has also been associated with poor sperm quality. It has been suggested that RF-EMF induce oxidative stress, leading to infertility.

Stress. Studies show that psychological stress can affect testosterone production, hormone balance and spermatogenesis. Stress has been linked to low sperm concentration, low motility and abnormal morphology.

Age and a decline in male fertility isn't a topic that gets much airtime, but it's an important consideration as age can affect male fertility in several ways. Excessive oxidative stress is associated with the ageing process. Accumulation of free radicals in male sperm cells throughout the course of ageing leads to oxidative stress and sperm DNA damage. As men grow older, testicular function and metabolism deteriorate and testosterone declines, leading to reduced sperm quality and quantity. Independent of maternal age, advanced paternal age has been associated with miscarriage and lower pregnancy rates amongst couples trying to conceive naturally and through IUI.

A large study looked at age thresholds for changes in semen parameters in men and found that parameters did not change before 34 years of age. But from 35 years of age, total sperm numbers and motility declined. Concentration and normal morphology declined after 40 years, motility and progressive parameters of motile

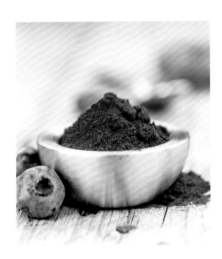

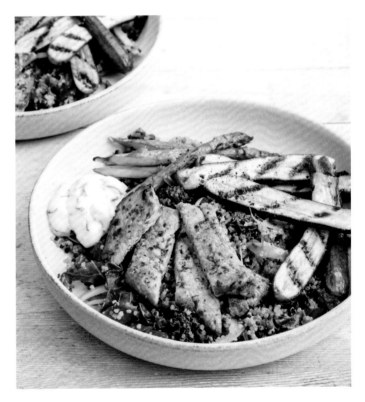

A diet rich in antioxidants supports sperm quality. Add blueberry powder to a smoothie (page 139) or make an Abundance bowl (pages 180–183) to boost antioxidant intake.

sperm fell after 43 years and ejaculate volume after 45 years.

Diet. Nutrition plays an important role in sperm quality. A diet rich in fish, chicken, fruit, vegetables, legumes and wholegrains has been associated with improved male fertility, while the standard 'Western' diet, characterised by a high intake of red and processed meat, refined grains, pizza, snacks, high-energy drinks and sweets, has been associated with poor semen quality.

Caffeine. It has been suggested that caffeine intake may negatively affect male fertility through sperm DNA damage, however, evidence on semen parameters and fertility is currently inconsistent and inconclusive. Most studies have reported no significant effects of moderate coffee consumption on semen quality. However, cola-containing beverages and caffeine-containing soft drinks have been associated with a negative effect on semen volume, count and concentration.

Environmental toxins. Multiple studies on exposure to environmental toxins suggest a negative impact on semen quality (concentration, motility and morphology). Metals and chemicals in air, water, food and health and beauty products may be damaging to fertility, affecting sperm count and function. The worst offenders are endocrine disrupters, which interfere with hormone balance. Phthalates, bisphenol A (BPA), dioxins and polychlorinated biphenyls (PCBs) are all associated with decreased semen quality and oxidative stress.

Optimising sperm quality

Eat through the rainbow to support intake of antioxidants, helping to offset free radicals. This is one of the most important things you can do to support male fertility. Use the Eat a rainbow tracker (pages 52–53) to help you identify colour gaps in your diet. Aim to eat a wide variety of vegetables to maximise intake of important antioxidant nutrients. Orange vegetables and fruits contain beta-carotene, an antioxidant associated with improved sperm concentration.

Balance blood sugar. High blood-sugar levels and insulin resistance are problematic for male fertility, and diets high in carbohydrates and sugar are associated with impaired sperm parameters. Insulin resistance is linked to inflammation and oxidative stress and is associated with lower testosterone levels and reduced sperm quality. Refer to blood-sugar balance (pages 22–26) and follow the recommendations to help balance your blood-sugar levels and optimise weight.

Optimise weight. Weight loss and lowering of BMI have been shown to improve sperm quality in some. The information in the Food pillar

Antioxidant boost

Add 1 teaspoon of wild blueberry powder (see Pantry staples on page 94) to a smoothie or yoghurt. One teaspoon of powder = one handful of fresh berries. Try Antioxidant burst soft serve (page 218) or A berry good start smoothie (page 139).

Smart supplements for sperm quality

Under the guidance of a nutritional therapist, consider the following supplements:

- ACETYL-L-CARNITINE has been shown to have a positive impact on sperm maturation, motility and spermatogenesis.
- ALPHA LIPOIC ACID is a powerful antioxidant, shown to improve sperm count, concentration and motility. Look for R-alpha lipoic acid, which is better utilised.
- COENZYME Q10 may support sperm quality due to its antioxidant effect and because it is involved in all energy-dependent processes, including sperm motility. Coenzyme Q10 has been linked to improved sperm count, motility, morphology and DNA integrity. Supplementation (in the form of ubiquinol) is recommended to help improve sperm quality as it is difficult to get optimal amounts from diet alone.
- LIPOSOMAL GLUTATHIONE is the mother of all antioxidants and protects sperm from oxidative stress during spermatogenesis and has been shown to improve sperm motility.
- MULTIVITAMIN. I recommend Pure Encapsulations O.N.E as it's a once-daily formula, which seems to improve compliance with men! A good-quality multivitamin contains a combination of nutrients and importantly, antioxidants, such as zinc. It is well established that taking a daily antioxidant supplement improves sperm quality.
- N-ACETYL CYSTEINE (NAC) is involved in glutathione synthesis and has powerful antioxidant properties. NAC has been associated with an increased number and motility of sperm as well as improved morphology and reduced DNA fragmentation.
- OMEGA-3 FATTY ACIDS. Sperm have a higher concentration of polyunsaturated fatty acids, and fertilisation depends on the lipid concentration of the sperm membrane. It has been demonstrated that omega-3 fats positively affect the concentration, number and morphology of sperm. Supplementation with the omega-3 fats EPA and DHA has been shown to significantly increase sperm motility and DHA concentration in semen and improve sperm DNA integrity. Supplementation is especially important if you do not eat oily fish, although aim to include this two to three times weekly as well (see pages 148–151 and 163–164 for recipes).

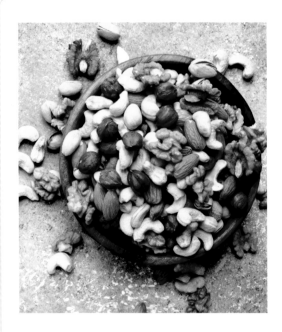

5 ways to add nuts to your diet

- Make a batch of homemade Granola (pages 140–141). Eat for breakfast or sprinkled on top of Overnight oats (page 134) or Oat bowls (pages 132–133).
- Add ground nuts to a smoothie (pages 138–139).
- Sprinkle whole nuts on top of soups, salads or curries.
- Serve mixed nuts and seeds or granola with berries and coconut yoghurt for dessert.
- Snack on a handful of nuts with carrot sticks, cucumber or celery.

(pages 48–97) will help you create a nutrient-rich diet that best supports fertility and weight management. The Fertility Kitchen plate (pages 72–74) is a useful tool for building balanced meals that help manage cravings and support satiety. This is particularly beneficial if you are transitioning from a standard Western diet.

Include nuts every day. Research shows the addition of just 60g (½ cup) nuts (almonds, hazelnuts and walnuts) daily to a Western-style diet significantly improves total sperm count and sperm vitality, motility and morphology. Nuts are a great source of vitamin E, and Brazil nuts are rich in selenium, both important antioxidant nutrients linked to improved male fertility.

Eat lycopene. Lycopene is the pigment that gives red tomatoes and some other red fruits and veg their vibrant colour. Lycopene is a phytonutrient with antioxidant properties that has been shown to improve sperm parameters such as concentration and motility. Lycopene in tomatoes increases during cooking, increasing antioxidant activity.

Limit alcohol intake. There is no definitive 'safe' level, so I recommend limiting to no more than two small glasses (125ml) of wine or 1–2 bottles of beer, depending on the strength, on a single occasion and no more than four times a week. Heavy alcohol consumption is linked to reduced sperm quality and increases oxidative stress, so take it easy! Organic red wine is a good choice as it contains the polyphenol resveratrol, which may have a protective effect on sperm function. Although this shouldn't be used as a reason to drink more – remember moderation is key!

Avoid trans fats such as margarine, vegetable oils and vegetable shortening,

5 ways to load up on lycopene

- Add sun-dried tomatoes to salad, Cauliflower pizza (page 174) or an Abundance bowl (pages 180–183).
- Spread tomato purée on Super-seedy crackers (page 146).
- Use my Failproof tomato sauce (page 208) as a base for curry, chilli or Bolognese.
- Try my Roasted Mediterranean veggie ragù (page 165) or Slow-cooker beef and black bean chilli (page 168).
- Enjoy roasted tomatoes with eggs for breakfast (page 126).

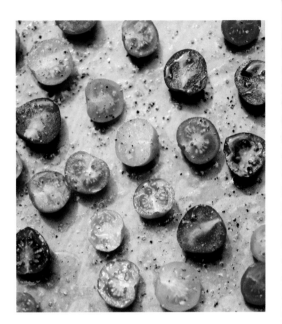

which are associated with poorer sperm quality and lower sperm concentration.

Avoid smoking. It is detrimental to male fertility, and the research is unequivocal. The same goes for recreational drugs.

Manage stress. Find ways to attenuate the stress in your life (pages 99–107).

Exercise to optimise your weight and help reduce oxidative stress. Moderate exercise *at least* three times weekly is ideal. Include strength training to support testosterone production. Increase your movement throughout the day, especially if you sit for prolonged periods of time, which may negatively affect fertility by raising scrotal temperature, as explained above (page 42).

Minimise exposure to environmental toxins from pollution, household and personal care products (see pages 112–116).

Keep your balls cool! Avoid keeping your smartphone in your trouser pocket, don't use a laptop directly on your lap, avoid prolonged sitting and other things that may increase scrotal temperature such as saunas, hot tubs or hot baths and tight underwear.

I hope the Fertility pillar has provided you with a deeper understanding of which factors might be influencing your fertility and given you the tools you need to start to take ownership of your reproductive health. The Food and Life pillars will help you to build on your plan and show you how to make simple, powerful and sustainable food and lifestyle changes to further support your fertility.

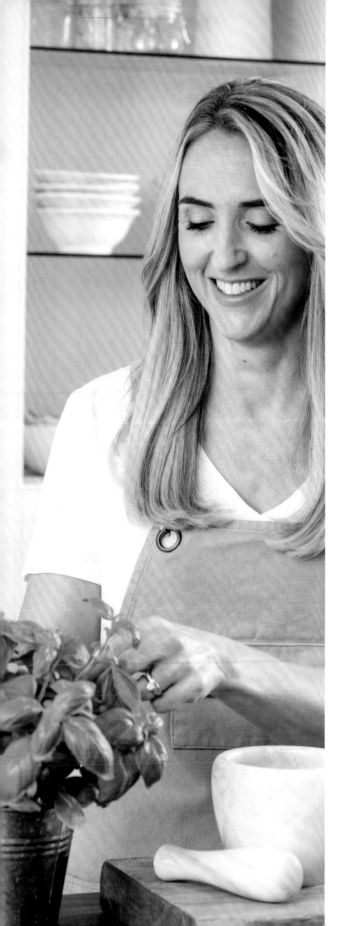

Food

The cornerstone of my approach is to support fertility primarily through a nutrient-rich, whole foods diet. This philosophy is about embracing foods in their natural state with an emphasis on food quality.

Your body runs on nutrients from food, so it makes sense that good-quality food should provide the foundation of your nutritional intake. Growing a baby is hard work, so by eating a nutrient-rich diet you will equip yourself with the building blocks your body needs to make a baby. Supplements are just that – supplements to real food.

Food is the most powerful ingredient to create optimal fertility – Charlotte Grand

Eat more plants

Make plants the foundation of your diet. The recipes I share make the most of seasonal vegetables, which have earned their place to be front and centre of your plate. This will naturally bring variety into your diet. When planning and cooking I encourage you to be flexible; follow the ebb and flow of the seasons and substitute the vegetables in the recipes accordingly.

For much of the year foods are not at their best, so eating with the seasons is such a treat and privilege. Vegetables taste superior in season when they are picked at their peak. They are also better for you as they are richer in nutrients. Fresh, local ingredients are key to a healthy, flavour-packed diet and there is almost always something good, fresh and locally produced for us all to enjoy.

Know your sources

Buying your food locally helps support your community and its farmers. You will know the origin of your food and be able to eat consciously. Quality of food is key and is especially important when buying meat and fish. Food writer Michael Pollan said it best: 'You are what you eat eats'.

Shop with integrity and favour organic, grass-fed meat, organic free-range poultry and eggs, and wild-caught fish. If you have a small budget for organic, this is where I urge you to prioritise. Buy humanely raised animals that have been fed their natural diet. Ensure that you can trace your food back to source.

If you can't find a suitable supplier locally, then consider using a vegetable box delivery service such as Riverford or Abel & Cole as you can also order good-quality meat and fish from these companies.

Top tip

Wash your fresh produce after purchase. Place fruits and vegetables in a bowl of filtered water with 2 tablespoons of apple cider vinegar. Let them soak for 10 minutes, then rinse with filtered water. Use a salad spinner or kitchen paper to dry them before storing in the fridge.

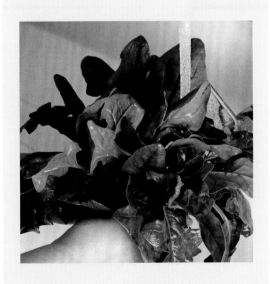

Go organic

The Fertility Kitchen recipes use organic ingredients. Switch to organic for reduced exposure to pesticides and toxic metals and increased nutrient density. If budget is an issue, look for organic frozen fruit and vegetables, which can be cheaper. Seasonal organic produce should also cost less than vegetables that are out of season. If your budget won't stretch to organic all the time, then prioritise buying the dirty dozen (most sprayed crops) organic and don't worry about the cleaner crops (see the Environmental Working Group's dirty dozen and clean fifteen in the table on the right). However, it's much better to eat vegetables than to avoid them because they're not organic, so if you can't justify the extra spend, then don't stress.

Make plants the foundation of your diet to increase nutrient density and diversity.

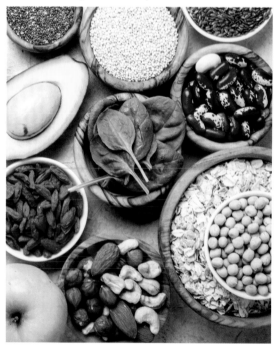

The dirty dozen and clean fifteen

Dirty dozen (most sprayed)	Cleanest 15 crops
Strawberries	Avocados
Spinach	Sweetcorn
Kale, collard and mustard greens	Pineapple (yay!)
Nectarines	Onions
Apples	Papaya
Grapes	Sweet peas (frozen)
Cherries	Aubergine
Peaches	Asparagus
Pears	Broccoli
Bell and hot peppers	Cabbage
Celery	Kiwi
Tomatoes	Cauliflower
	Mushrooms
	Honeydew melon
	Cantaloupe

Fertility-friendly food habits

Eat dense

This simply means choosing foods that have a nutrient-rich profile (more bang for your buck!). For example, a plate of vegetables contains an abundance of vitamins and minerals, whereas a plate of refined pasta does not. Nutrient-rich foods best support fertility and overall health. Remember that normal bodily processes such as detoxification require a lot of nutrients for optimal function. If your dietary intake of vital nutrients is low, your body will prioritise these essential functions over your fertility.

The nutrient density of your meals can be affected by food selection, storage and cooking. Eat fresh vegetables abundantly and enjoy them as soon as you can after purchase – the longer they are stored, the more nutrients they lose. Eat a variety of cooked and raw vegetables and don't forget to make use of your freezer. Frozen vegetables are typically picked ripe and flash-frozen to preserve their nutrition. They can be a better choice than fresh, which quickly lose nutrients. You can also buy ready-chopped frozen vegetables and herbs, which makes life easier. Frozen seafood tends to be more affordable than fresh, which is a bonus!

Ignore the ick factor and include organ meat in your diet. You can easily hide this in recipes (pages 168 and 178). Prioritise seafood, which is incredibly nutrient dense. If you like nuts and seeds, favour Brazil nuts, and pumpkin, sesame and sunflower seeds, which are the most nutrient-rich of the bunch.

Eat the rainbow

A healthy food pattern is diverse, varied and colourful. Eating the rainbow is a game-changer at helping you to get all the nutrients that you and your future baby need to thrive. It's as straightforward as eating all the colours of the rainbow every day and aiming for variety: 30 different plants over the course of a week. We're all guilty of falling into the trap of buying the same vegetables and fruits week-in, week-out. It's time to step out of your comfort zone and be adventurous with ingredients and recipes. Make a pizza base out of cauliflower (page 174), noodles out of courgette (page 142) and rice out of vegetables (pages 195–197). The recipes in this book will inspire you to expand your vegetable repertoire.

Use the Eat a rainbow tracker on pages 52–53 to help keep track of your colour intake throughout the week. To download a copy to print out and complete, see page 233. If you're missing any colours, list different vegetables and fruits to include in your diet to plug the gaps. An easy solution is to try veg at breakfast, (see pages 126 and 129–130 for veggie-based breakfast recipes or head to pages 184–199 for veg inspiration).

Did you know?

Liver also goes by the name of 'nature's multivitamin' because it is so abundant in nutrients. My top tip is to freeze it and then grate it into your cooking. Add to sauces, curries and chilli for an extra nutrient hit.

Eat a rainbow tracker

	Green	White	Yellow
	Green apple, artichoke, asparagus, avocado, green beans, beet greens, pak choi, broccoli, Brussels sprouts, Savoy cabbage, Romanesco cauliflower, cavolo nero, celery, collard greens, courgette, cucumber, edamame beans, endive, kale, kiwi, romaine lettuce, okra, olives, garden peas, green peppers, rocket, spinach, Swiss chard, watercress	Jerusalem artichokes, white cabbage, cauliflower, coconut, fennel, garlic, lychees, mushrooms, onions, parsnips, white peaches, pears, shallots, turnips, yams	Cantaloupe, root ginger, grapefruit, lemons, peaches, yellow pepper, pineapple, summer squash, sweetcorn
MON			
TUES			
WED			
THUR			
FRI			
SAT			
SUN			

Apricots, butternut squash, carrots, mangoes, oranges, papaya, orange pepper, pumpkin, sweet potato, tangerine, turmeric root, yellow carrots	Red apples, beetroot, blood orange, cranberries, cherries, red grapes, nectarines, red onions, red peppers, pomegranates, radicchio, radish, raspberries, rhubarb, strawberries, tomatoes	Aubergine, blueberries, blackberries, purple broccoli, red cabbage, purple carrots, purple cauliflower, elderberries, figs, black grapes, purple kale, kalamata olives, plums, purple sweet potato

The 90/10 approach

This approach is about moving away from the idea of being 'on a diet' or 'falling off the wagon' and 'getting back on track'. It's a way of life, so include foods such as sweet treats, for the sheer joy of eating them. Make them an occasional part of your life if you want them to be. I like to think of them as mindful indulgences, which removes the stress and the guilt and makes eating to optimise your fertility sustainable. You don't have to give up everything you enjoy; strive to eat well at least 90 per cent of the time and eat what you fancy the rest of the time. This could be a meal out or a glass of good-quality red wine with dinner at the weekend. It's not 'bad', it's part of enjoying life.

Many of my clients have found it helpful to work on their mindset when it comes to thinking about foods that are best avoided. Instead of thinking 'I can't eat that', which almost always leads to constantly thinking about that particular food, try saying 'I can eat that, but I choose not to'. This subtle shift is simple but empowering and will help you adjust to a new way of eating for life.

Try this

Head to pages 210–223 and pick one of my sweet recipes. Make whichever sweet appeals the most, then sit down with your favourite brew and take the time to really savour it. I guarantee this will feel so much more enjoyable than mindlessly stuffing your face while watching TV and then wondering how you managed to eat an entire packet of biscuits!

It's all about perspective

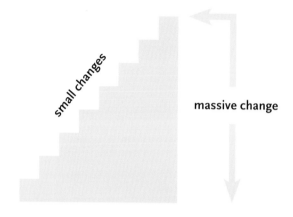

small changes

massive change

Progress over perfection

My favourite mantra! Eating is meant to be a pleasure and turning your whole diet upside-down in one go is no fun for anyone. Instead focus on small, consistent changes. Be realistic and accomplish one change before moving on to the next.

I love this quote:

When nothing seems to help, I go and look at a stonecutter hammering away at his rock perhaps a hundred times without as much as a crack showing in it. Yet at the hundred-and-first blow it will split in two, and I know that it was not the last blow that did it – but all that had gone before. Jacob Riis

This is so apt for changing your diet to support your fertility. It highlights the importance of progress over perfection. Be patient and keep going, even without a positive pregnancy test. Your hard work is not wasted, you are building on small, important changes to your diet every day, which amounts to a lot over time. Recognise other positive changes to your health and wellbeing that you can use as a gauge for the impact your diet and lifestyle changes are making, rather than only focusing on your goal of pregnancy.

Fertility nutrition foundations

The macronutrients are the cornerstone nutrients that we get from food. We need them in larger quantities, and they play a central role in tissue formation and energy production. Optimal fertility nutrition relies upon a healthy balance of all three major macronutrients: carbohydrates, protein and fat.

Carbohydrates

Carbohydrates provide you with a quick energy source (glucose) and are the preferred fuel source for the brain. They help to regulate fat and protein metabolism and provide fibre to support gut health. Many people eat too much of the wrong type of carbohydrates. There are two broad categories, based on the way we digest them and their impact on our blood sugar:

- Simple carbohydrates (sugar, refined flour, sweets, etc.) have many sugar (glucose) molecules strung together in simple structures. These are very easy to digest and so result in a quick and significant rise in blood sugar.
- Complex carbohydrates (vegetables, wholegrains, legumes) have their sugar molecules arranged in more complex structures and are also woven with indigestible fibres. These are harder to digest and so result in a slower and more moderate rise in blood sugar. However, this can depend on how much we eat and in what combination.

Break up with refined carbohydrates

Refined carbohydrates do not serve your fertility. Limit or ideally avoid the following:

- Refined grains and all products made from white flour: bread, bagels, cereals, crackers, crisps, noodles, pasta, pastries, popcorn, rice cakes, white rice and the like.
- All forms of added sugar (check food labels carefully as sugar has over 70 different names – see page 232 for the full list and page 25 for information on understanding food labels).

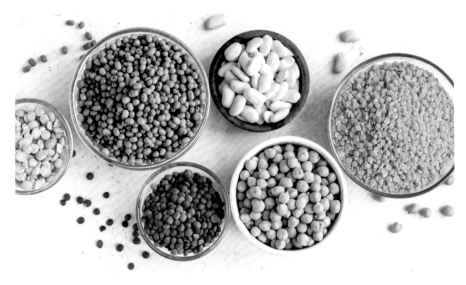

Legumes are a source of complex carbohydrate.

- Sweetened drinks, including soft drinks, squash and fruit juice.
- Artificial sugars and sweeteners, including diet soft drinks and sugar-free squash.

Generally, the more refined carbohydrates you eat, the less nutritious your diet overall. I know avoiding refined carbs can feel overwhelming, but keep your goal in mind. Remember that you're in the right hands and that I've got you covered with a wealth of ideas, flavours and tastes to inspire you.

You can't cheat sweet

In general, your body can cope with modest sugar consumption – think occasionally, not every day. However, I do live in the real world and I know that it takes a rare woman to completely avoid the sweet stuff (I'm yet to meet her!). So, you'll note that I've included some yummy better-for-you sweet recipes (pages 210–223). If you absolutely must add sweetener to something, use only a small amount (¼–½ tsp) of date syrup, coconut syrup, honey or maple syrup. My preferred sweetener is raw or manuka honey.

Truth bomb

Dried fruit is not a healthy sweet. It is extremely concentrated in sugar. A snack box size of raisins has over 29g of sugar – that's more than 7 teaspoons!

GRAINS: Swap this for that

Try replacing the grains on your plate with vegetables:

INSTEAD OF PASTA made from refined flour → Try courgette noodles (page 142).

INSTEAD OF A PIZZA BASE made from refined flour → Try a cauliflower pizza base (page 174).

INSTEAD OF WHITE RICE → Maximise your veg intake with veggie rice (pages 195–197).

What carbs *can* you eat?

The best carbohydrates you can eat to support fertility are non-starchy vegetables (artichoke, asparagus, aubergine, Batavia lettuce, bell pepper, broccoli, butterhead lettuce, Brussels sprouts, cabbage, cauliflower, carrots, cavolo nero, celery, collard greens, cos lettuce, courgette, cucumber, endive, garlic, iceberg, kale, mushrooms, onions, pea shoots, radish, rocket, spinach, spring onions, Swiss chard, watercress). These have minimal impact on blood sugar and are rich in nutrients and fibre. You can go crazy with these! Low sugar, whole fruits (berries, citrus, green apples, tomatoes and avocado) are also fabulous. Enjoy 1–2 portions a day (see page 72–74 for portion guidance).

You can include starchy vegetables (parsnips, potatoes, squash and sweet potatoes) and legumes in your diet as they offer wonderful nutrition. I consider wholegrains to be nutritionally underwhelming; you can include them, but they won't be missed if you choose not to (unless you are vegan), and some people feel better without them. Eat this category in moderation because large quantities can still have a significant impact on your blood sugar, especially if eaten on their own. Limit to one type with each meal and enjoy as a smaller side dish portion (see pages 72–74 for more on this).

Size guide

You probably need far fewer carbohydrates than you realise. I recommend a low-to-moderate intake of around 20–40 per cent of your daily calories – we all have different requirements, with some needing more and others less. How much *you* need depends on many factors such as your weight, blood-sugar handling, activity level, genetics and whether you have any hormonal conditions, such as polycystic ovary syndrome (PCOS).

Take an intuitive approach

Start at 20 per cent of your daily calories and monitor how you feel. If you find you are low on energy, then increase your serving size of starchy vegetables, legumes or wholegrains. Conversely, if you are eating closer to 40 per cent and you experience headaches, dizziness or irritability between meals, then it's a good idea to reduce your serving size. The key is to start tuning into your body – symptoms are your body's way of communicating that something isn't quite right. Pay attention.

Include an abundance of non-starchy vegetables in your diet.

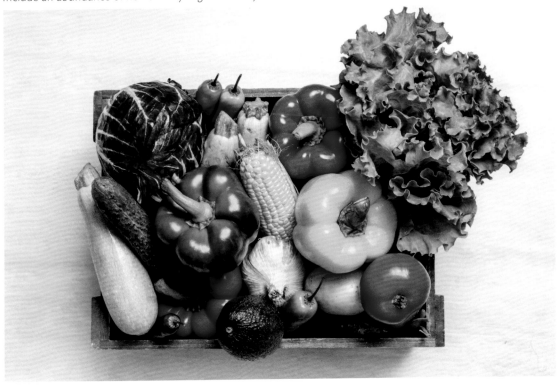

Carbs at a glance

Load up on	Eat moderately	Limit	Avoid
• Non-starchy vegetables	• Starchy vegetables • Wholegrains • Legumes • Low-sugar whole fruits	• Sweet whole fruit (banana, pineapple, mango, figs, grapes) • Dried fruit • Sugar in the form of coconut sugar or syrup, date syrup, honey, maple syrup	• Added sugar • Anything made from refined flour (bread, pasta, crackers, pastries, cookies, cereals, crisps) • Artificial sugars and sweeteners • Sweetened drinks and fruit juice

You can use an app (such as Cronometer or MyFitnessPal) to help you get started, but I don't recommend obsessively tracking your macronutrients. The Fertility Kitchen plate (pages 72–74) is a simple tool that you can use as a guide to visually plan your meals. If you follow this, then tracking won't be necessary. If you feel that you need additional support or guidance, I suggest working with a nutritional therapist (see Resources on page 235).

If you will be cutting back your carbohydrate intake considerably (e.g., if you are transitioning from a Western-style diet), ensure that you're increasing your intake of protein and healthy fat at the same time. Otherwise, you are unlikely to feel full or satisfied. Including protein and fat at every meal is also important to support blood-sugar balance and maintain steady energy levels throughout the day. Read more on pages 22–26.

Protein

Protein is fundamental for optimal health and fertility. Its component amino acids provide the building blocks for your body and that of your future baby. Protein is particularly critical in the first and third trimesters of pregnancy. As well as being important for your growing baby, it also allows your body to adapt to pregnancy.

Protein provides the raw materials to make certain hormones, antibodies, enzymes, neurotransmitters, and haemoglobin (which delivers oxygen throughout your body in your blood). For fertility, protein is important for healthy hormones, your menstrual cycle, immune system, thyroid health and detoxification.

Complete vs incomplete

Amino acids are the building blocks of protein. Twenty amino acids are used to build the proteins in your body, nine of

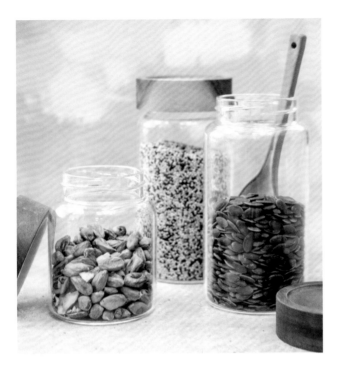

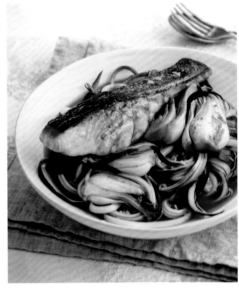

Protein is crucial for optimal fertility. Include a wide variety of animal and plant protein in your diet.

which are considered essential. The nine essential amino acids are: histidine, isoleucine, leucine, lysine, methionine, phenylalanine, threonine, tryptophan and valine. You must get these nine from food as your body can't make them, whereas it can make the other eleven. Six of these eleven are considered conditionally essential, meaning their synthesis can be limited under certain conditions. The remaining five amino acids are nutritionally dispensable, meaning that you don't need to get them from food. However, for optimal health and fertility, it is far preferable to get all twenty amino acids from food.

Complete proteins deliver enough of all nine essential amino acids and are mostly animal foods (meat, poultry, eggs, seafood and dairy), with only a few exceptions. Animal proteins also contain all twenty amino acids so when you eat these foods your body doesn't have to rely on inefficient conversion processes for the amino acids it needs to make its various protein types. On the other hand, most plant foods are incomplete proteins and will be missing at least one of the nine essential amino acids. If you follow a vegan diet you will need to consciously eat a variety of plant foods to ensure that you are getting the full spectrum of amino acids needed to make complete proteins.

However, plant proteins can be problematic for your body to digest, while all animal proteins (especially seafood) are easier to digest. This doesn't mean that plants aren't incredibly important for health, simply that it is misleading to regard them as a superior protein source.

I recommend including seafood in your fertility diet at the very least, if not a wide variety of animal foods. Studies have found that eating fish significantly improves fertility in both men and women.

Protein at a glance

Best-quality protein	Best plant protein*	Best avoided
• Wild-caught fish and seafood • Organic free-range poultry and eggs • Grass-fed red meats • Organic liver and bone broth • Organic full-fat dairy (if tolerated) • High-quality protein powders (e.g. grass-fed collagen, pure marine collagen, organic grass-fed pure whey protein)	• Beans and legumes (aduki beans, black beans, borlotti beans, butter beans, chickpeas, kidney beans, lentils, mung beans, pinto beans, split lentils) • Nuts (almonds, Brazil nuts, cashews, hazelnuts, macadamia nuts, peanuts, pecans, pistachios, walnuts) • Seeds (chia seeds, flaxseeds, hemp seeds, pumpkin seeds, sesame seeds, sunflower seeds) • Wholegrains and pseudo grains (amaranth, buckwheat, brown and wild rice, oats, quinoa) • High-quality organic plant protein powder (check ingredients)	• Deli and processed meats (bacon, canned meat, chorizo, corned beef, dried meat, ham, hot dogs, pancetta, prosciutto, salami, salted and cured meat, sausages, smoked meat) • Meat replacements (fake, faux or mock meats made from mycoprotein, textured vegetable protein (or textured soy protein), seitan (sometimes called wheat gluten, wheat protein or wheat meat) • Soy products (textured vegetable protein, tofu and non-organic tempeh) • Most commercial protein powders

*Legumes, nuts, seeds and grains are not complete proteins (except for buckwheat, chia seeds, hemp seeds and quinoa). If you're vegetarian or vegan, be mindful of eating a variety of plant protein sources (both legumes and wholegrains or pseudo grains) every day to provide your body with the full complement of amino acids it needs to function.

Size guide

Everyone is different. Start at around 20 per cent of your daily calories and adjust up or down as needed, based on how you feel. As a general guide, make protein a palm-sized participant on your plate (see The Fertility Kitchen plate on pages 72–74).

The UK recommended daily intake of protein is set at 0.75g of protein per kilogram bodyweight. This amounts to 51g for a woman weighing 68kg. However, keep in mind that this is considered a minimum daily allowance.

A recent study that directly measured protein requirements during pregnancy found that a 68kg woman needed 83g of protein per day in the first trimester, jumping to 105g per day in the third trimester. This demonstrates the importance of protein in pregnancy. Make sure that you are meeting these additional needs when you do become pregnant.

Soaking legumes and wholegrains

Legumes and wholegrains contain higher levels of phytic acid and digestive enzyme inhibitors that may impair digestion in some people (ever noticed bloating after eating beans?). Preparation techniques can improve their digestibility, making their nutrients easier to absorb. Find my easy soaking and cooking guide in the Appendix on pages 230–231.

Fat

For far too long fat has been unfairly demonised. A lot of women are still actively avoiding fat. If that's you too, it's time to reframe your thinking and embrace healthy fat. Fat is hugely important for optimal health and fertility. It provides a concentrated energy source and is important for hormone production, nutrient absorption and blood-sugar regulation. There are many different fatty acids (the building blocks of fat) and you need balanced amounts of each.

Saturated fatty acids

Saturated fats are easy for your body to digest and use for energy and are important for sex hormone production, brain health, cell membrane structure and immune health. They are stable and not easily oxidised (meaning that they aren't susceptible to react chemically with oxygen). This makes them a great choice for high-temperature cooking such as roasting. Saturated fats can be found in animal and plant foods such as butter and ghee, full-fat dairy, lard and coconut oil. Use sparingly for cooking and spreading.

Monounsaturated fatty acids

Monounsaturated fats are anti-inflammatory and important for immune health, healthy

How much protein do you need?

To calculate the right protein intake for your bodyweight:

1.22g of protein per kg bodyweight (first trimester)

1.52g of protein per kg bodyweight (third trimester)

cholesterol levels and insulin sensitivity. Monounsaturated fats are less stable than saturated fat and require more enzymes to break them apart in order to be used as energy. Good sources include avocados, avocado oil, macadamia nuts, olives and olive oil. Olive oil contains oleic acid, the main fat found in developing egg cells and plays an important role in egg development.

Polyunsaturated fatty acids

Polyunsaturated fatty acids are also known as essential fatty acids and are broadly categorised into omega-3 and omega-6 fatty acids.

Omega-3 fatty acids are anti-inflammatory and are important for cell membrane function, immune health, sperm and egg health, and your baby's brain development. The three most important omega-3 fatty acids are:

- **Alpha-linolenic acid (ALA)**
- **Eicosapentaenoic acid (EPA)**
- **Docosahexaenoic acid (DHA)**

Of these fats, only ALA is officially deemed essential (meaning you must get it from food). This is because your body can make EPA and DHA from ALA. This is somewhat misleading because the conversion process can be very inefficient, so it is important to get all *three* from food. ALA is abundant in plant foods such as chia seeds, flaxseeds, flaxseed oil, walnuts and walnut oil. EPA and DHA are abundant in seafood (especially fatty cold-water fish), grass-fed meat, free-range poultry and eggs. Women with a sufficient level of omega-3 fats have been shown to have higher-quality embryos in IVF and a higher chance of conceiving.

Omega-6 fatty acids are important for cell membrane function and energy production. They are only needed in small amounts. The most important omega-6 fatty acids are:

- **Linoleic acid (LA)**
- **Arachidonic acid (AA)**

Only LA is deemed essential (meaning you must get it from food) because your body can make AA from LA. However, the conversion process can be inefficient here too, so you need to get *both* from food. LA has been linked to improved fertility and can be found in nuts and seeds. AA is found in meat, poultry and eggs.

The polyunsaturated fatty acids (nuts, seeds and their oils) are prone to oxidation, which means that they react chemically with oxygen very easily. This reaction breaks the fatty acid apart and produces oxidants. In turn, eating these damaged fats causes

What to look for in an olive oil

- **Quality is key: a good olive oil will have a pungent flavour.**
- **Choose extra virgin and avoid refined.**
- **Fresh is best! Olive oil won't improve with age – look for a harvest date on the bottle (the more recent, the better).**
- **Look for dark glass bottles (never clear or plastic) and store in a cool, dark cupboard.**
- **Buy a smaller bottle so that you can finish it while it's still fresh (even a high-quality oil stored correctly will start to degrade after a few months).**

oxidative stress in the body and this can harm fertility.

Balancing your intake of omega-3 and omega-6 fatty acids

It is important to balance your intake of omega-3 and omega-6 fatty acids. A healthy ratio is somewhere in the range of 1:1 and 1:4 – this is the ratio at which your body does best. Shockingly, the ratio of a typical Western diet has been found to be between 1:10 and 1:30!

To balance your intake of these fats you will need to be mindful about lowering your intake of omega-6 (abundant in grains, industrially produced meat, legumes, nuts, seeds and vegetable oils) while increasing your intake of the important omega-3s DHA and EPA (found predominantly in seafood, especially oily fish). Be conscientious about including seafood in your fertility diet.

Fats to avoid

Steer clear of processed vegetable oils and trans fats. These are the worst fats that you can eat. Vegetable oils need to be extensively processed because they don't give up their fats easily. This processing includes chemical treatment, high heat and toxic solvents. These oils are very susceptible to oxidation and consuming them is detrimental to your health. Trans fats are vegetable oils that have been hydrogenated. The highest levels of trans fats are found in margarines, processed snack foods, frozen dinners and fast food. Vegetable oils also hide in plant milks and hummus. But don't worry, it's incredibly easy to make your own (pages 137 and 200–201).

Top tip

Store nuts and seeds in an airtight container in the fridge. Look for nut and seed oils (e.g. flaxseed, sesame and walnut oils) in dark glass bottles and store them in the fridge. Use within six months. You will know if nuts, seeds and their oils have oxidised as they will smell rancid.

Ditch these unhealthy fats...

Vegetable oils (canola, corn, cooking sprays, cottonseed, grape seed, palm kernel, peanut, safflower, soybean, sunflower, vegetable), margarine and other butter substitutes, shortening and anything with hydrogenation or partial hydrogenation on the label.

...and use these healthy fats instead

Fat makes your food tastes good! I love to stir-fry and bake with a little olive oil or coconut oil; you can also use ghee and butter. I use avocado and extra virgin olive oil to drizzle over salads and veggies. Check out my favourite dressings on pages 204–207.

Fats at a glance

Saturated	Monounsaturated	Polyunsaturated	Fats to avoid
Use sparingly for cooking at high temperatures:	Use for cooking, dressing, drizzling or garnishing:	Include as your protein source or use for flavouring and garnishing:	• Hydrogenated (trans fats) • Margarine • Vegetable oils • Vegetable shortening
• Butter and ghee • Lard • Coconut oil	• Avocados • Avocado oil • Nuts and seeds, esp. macadamia nuts • Olives and olive oil	**Omega-3** Focus on DHA and EPA from: • Oily fish (2–3 times weekly) • Seaweed (nori, kelp, wakame) • Free-range egg yolks (1–2 daily)	
Use sparingly as a flavour highlight: • Full-fat dairy		**Omega-6** Focus on LA from: • Nuts • Seeds	

Size guide

Again, everyone's needs will be different, and a wide range of between 30–60 per cent of daily calories can be healthy. The key is to focus on a balanced and varied intake of each of the fatty acids. Listen to your body and consider symptoms such as poor energy, digestive upset or hormone imbalance as a sign that you may need to adjust your fat intake.

Avocado is a good source of monounsaturated fat.

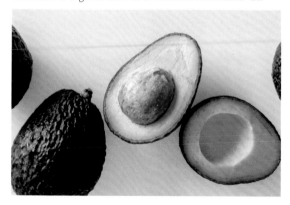

The fertility micronutrient hotlist

Micronutrients are required in smaller amounts and include vitamins, minerals and phytonutrients. They are nutritional superstars – every minute element of every function of every part of your body requires them. Even slight deficiency can have a negative impact on your fertility.

Load up on these vitamins and minerals to supercharge your fertility:

Nutrient	Important for	Top food sources
Preformed vitamin A (retinol)	Sperm and egg cell development and maturation, fertilisation, foetal development	Liver, meat, poultry, high-quality dairy products, seafood
Vitamin B6	Methylation and gene regulation, detoxification and enzyme reactions, blood-sugar balance, immune function, mental health, essential to produce the corpus luteum and support the luteal phase, foetal brain development	Leafy and root vegetables, fruits such as bananas, red meat, poultry, seeds (sunflower and pumpkin)
Vitamin B9 (folate)	Methylation and gene regulation, prevents neural tube defects	Liver, green vegetables, legumes, beetroot, avocados
Vitamin B12	Female fertility, sperm quality, foetal development, preventing miscarriage, methylation and gene regulation	Seafood, liver, red meat, poultry, eggs
Calcium	Healthy bones and teeth, egg and embryo development, fertilisation and implantation, prevents clots and preeclampsia, foetal development	Dark-green leafy vegetables, sesame seeds, dairy, whole sardines, squash

Nutrient	Important for	Top food sources
Choline	Foetal brain development, placental function, helps prevent neural tube defects	Seafood, liver, eggs (yolks), poultry, green veggies
Vitamin D	Deficiency is associated with infertility, PCOS, endometriosis, early pregnancy loss, preeclampsia, gestational diabetes, preterm birth, thyroid dysfunction	Oily fish, mushrooms, fish roe, liver, eggs
DHA	Egg health and sperm quality, immune health and lowering inflammation, foetal brain and eye development	Fatty fish such as salmon, Atlantic mackerel, herring, sardines

Your body makes vitamin D from sun exposure. Spend as much time outside as you can.

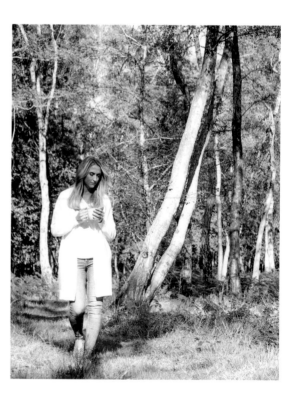

Soak up the sunshine

Get outside and enjoy 15–30 minutes of sunshine a day for that all-important vitamin D hit. Sunlight exposure accounts for 90 per cent of vitamin D in the body in those who do not supplement.

Nutrient	Important for	Top food sources
Iodine	Low levels linked to hypothyroidism and infertility and demand increases during pregnancy	Sea vegetables (especially kelp and wakame), seafood, eggs, dairy
Iron	Reduces the risk of ovulatory infertility, builds red blood cells, deficiency causes anaemia. Important for liver detoxification and healthy thyroid function.	Liver, red meat, dark-green leafy vegetables, legumes
Vitamin K2	Insulin sensitivity and blood-sugar control, early embryo development, calcium use and strong bones for you and your baby	Natto, eggs, butter, liver
Magnesium	Blood sugar and blood pressure, enzyme reactions and detox, energy and protein production, reduces pre-term labour risk	Green vegetables, nuts and seeds, fish, legumes, avocados
Selenium	Sperm health, female fertility, immune health, antioxidative activities, deficiency linked with miscarriage, healthy thyroid	Red meat, poultry, seafood, Brazil nuts, mushrooms
Zinc	Male fertility, female fertility, fertilisation and embryo growth, sex hormone production and metabolism, thyroid hormone conversion, lowering inflammation	Oysters, red meat, poultry, nuts, seeds, legumes

Plant-based eating and fertility: what you need to know

There are several nutrients vital for fertility that are either difficult or impossible to obtain in sufficient amounts from plants alone. These are: preformed vitamin A (retinol), vitamin B12, choline, DHA, glycine, iron, vitamin K2 and zinc.

IMPOSSIBLE: move straight to the chart on page 69	DIFFICULT: read on to learn why
Preformed vitamin A, vitamin B12	Choline, DHA, glycine, iron, vitamin K2, zinc

Choline

The richest sources of choline are egg yolks and liver. Although some plant foods do contain choline (e.g. certain cruciferous vegetables), the relative concentration is far less than the richest animal sources, making it challenging to meet your needs. Egg-eaters have roughly double the intake of choline than non-egg-eaters. If you are avoiding eggs, you are unlikely to get enough of this nutrient.

DHA

Algae is the only noteworthy plant source of DHA. I'm yet to come across someone who chows down on this at all, let alone in the quantity that would be required to meet your nutrient needs!

Glycine

The relative concentration of glycine in plant foods compared to animal foods is very low. Top plant foods include sesame seed flour, spirulina algae, pumpkin seeds, nori (seaweed), watercress, beans and spinach. However, you are unlikely to get enough.

Iron and zinc

Although iron and zinc aren't exclusively found in animal foods, the difficulty lies in absorption of these nutrients from plant foods.

There are two forms of dietary iron: heme and non-heme. Heme iron, found only in animal foods such as red meat, poultry and seafood, is well absorbed; while non-heme iron, found in plants, is less well absorbed. Over 95 per cent of the iron in our bodies is in the form of heme iron. To find out if you are deficient, evaluate your iron status by testing your ferritin level either via your GP or an online blood-testing service (see Resources on page 235).

Zinc is also found in both animal foods (red meat and seafood) and plants (nuts, seeds and legumes), and like iron, is less well absorbed from plants. It is difficult to obtain sufficient iron and zinc from plants alone.

Vitamin K2

This vitamin is only found in animal foods (such as liver, beef and chicken) and fermented plant foods. Natto is a rich plant source, but I've never met anyone who eats this! Natto is a traditional Japanese food made from fermented soybeans and has a sticky texture and distinctive taste that has been likened to old Brie. If you can get hold of this, 1 tablespoon contains about 300mcg of vitamin K2. Sauerkraut may also provide vitamin K2, however, it would be difficult to

Smart supplements for plant-based diets

Nutrient	Supplement info
Vitamin A – while your body can convert beta-carotene into vitamin A, conversion is inefficient	Your prenatal multivitamin should contain both preformed vitamin A and beta-carotene. Ensure that you do not exceed 5000 IU of preformed vitamin A daily as this may result in toxicity
Vitamin B12	300mcg per day in the form of methylcobalamin and/or adenosylcobalamin. It's likely that your prenatal multivitamin won't have enough
Choline	450–930mg. Look for choline bitartrate or sunflower lecithin (phosphatidylcholine)
DHA	Look for an algae-based DHA supplement
Glycine	The minimum amount of glycine needed in the diet is 10g per day (for non-pregnant adults; this increases in pregnancy)
Iron	Around 27mg per day, but this will depend on your current level (check ferritin levels via your GP or online blood-testing service – see Resources on page 235)
Vitamin K2	100mcg per day from a separate supplement
Zinc	Ensure that your prenatal multivitamin has at least 11mg

eat enough to meet your needs. Your gut bacteria are also capable of synthesising vitamin K2 in small amounts, but this depends on optimal gut health.

What can you do about it?

Supplementation is fundamental for you to meet your nutrient needs for optimal fertility and pregnancy. You'll need to check how much of each nutrient is in your prenatal multivitamin and look to add in extras to plug the gaps (see table on page 69). If you follow a vegan diet, it is worth seeking the help of a nutritional therapist to ensure that you are meeting your nutrient needs to fully support fertility and a healthy pregnancy.

Hydration

You won't be surprised to learn that water should be your number-one drink of choice. Your body loses water consistently through urine, breath, sweat and stool, so it's vital to replenish frequently. Aim for about 2.2 litres a day, including all drinks and the water you get from food, which makes up to 20 per cent of your daily water intake. Quality of water is key, and I recommend filtering it (page 114).

Try healthy vitamin water instead of plain water (see box opposite).

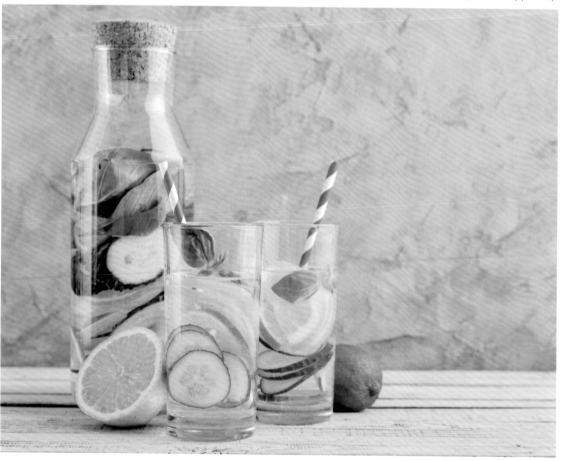

The limit list

Alcohol

- Limit to one small drink (e.g. one small glass (125ml) of organic red wine) per occasion (women) while trying to conceive; for men, one to two drinks per occasion (e.g. two small glasses (125ml) of organic red wine, or one to two bottles of beer, depending on the strength) and no more than four alcoholic drinks per week (both partners).
- If you choose to drink, consider an occasional small glass (125ml) of organic red wine with dinner (this could be your mindful indulgence at the weekend, see page 54). Red wine contains resveratrol, an antioxidant compound that has potential therapeutic effects for improving ovarian function and male fertility.
- Ideally keep alcohol intake to an absolute minimum and avoid for best results!
- Not safe in pregnancy; even small amounts have been shown to be harmful, so avoid completely when you do get pregnant. Some women prefer to avoid alcohol during the luteal phase of their cycle in case they are pregnant.

Caffeine

- Heavy caffeine consumption (four or more cups per day), even before pregnancy, has been linked with an increased risk of miscarriage.
- A lower intake may still increase miscarriage risk, which is reported to rise at 50–150mg per day during pregnancy.
- 1 cup of coffee contains 100–200mg, black tea contains about 50mg and green tea 25mg per cup.
- 1 cup of tea or half a cup of coffee per day is safest, or switch to decaffeinated.
- If you choose to drink coffee, try the brand Lean Caffeine, which does not contain pesticides, heavy metals or mycotoxins.
- Pay attention to your body – if you experience headaches, jitteriness or anxiety after consumption, then it's best avoided.
- Avoid caffeinated soft drinks and energy drinks.
- Consider avoiding caffeine completely during IVF and once you become pregnant.

The Fertility Kitchen plate

The Fertility Kitchen plate is a quick and easy method for creating a balanced meal, without needing to strictly measure portions.

What does a balanced meal look like?

Fill half your plate with non-starchy vegetables

- Eat the rainbow (see Eat a rainbow tracker on pages 52–53 for help with this).
- Aim for eight portions of vegetables every day. Measuring cups (page 97) are an easy way to measure vegetable portion sizes as 1 cup = 1 portion. Strive to include 2 cups at breakfast, 3 cups at lunch and 3 cups at dinner. Aim to vary vegetable types: 3 cups = 1 cup of cruciferous vegetables (broccoli, Brussels sprouts, cabbage, cauliflower, collard greens, kale, rocket and watercress), 1 cup of leafy greens (beet greens, collard greens, cabbage, endive, kale, microgreens, romaine lettuce, Swiss chard, pak choi, rocket and watercress) and 1 cup of brightly coloured vegetables. Some vegetables are both cruciferous and leafy green, so just choose two different ones.
- Eat fresh, raw or lightly cooked.
- Use healthy fats, herbs and spices to flavour your vegetables.
- Consume vegetables and fruit in a ratio of 4:1 – see (pages 52–53) for fruit recommendations.

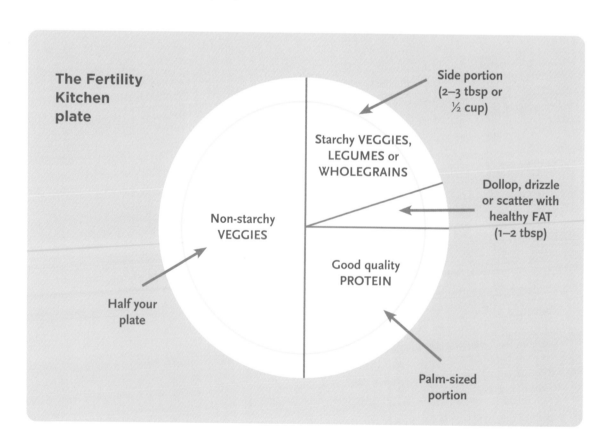

The Fertility Kitchen plate

Half your plate

Non-starchy VEGGIES

Starchy VEGGIES, LEGUMES or WHOLEGRAINS

Good quality PROTEIN

Side portion (2–3 tbsp or ½ cup)

Dollop, drizzle or scatter with healthy FAT (1–2 tbsp)

Palm-sized portion

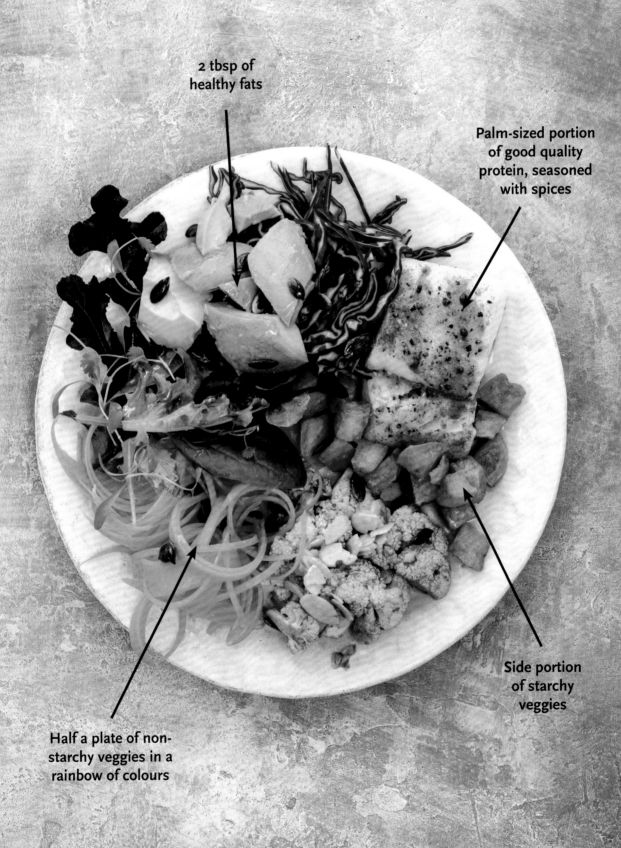

2 tbsp of
healthy fats

Palm-sized portion
of good quality
protein, seasoned
with spices

Side portion
of starchy
veggies

Half a plate of non-
starchy veggies in a
rainbow of colours

Add a palm-sized portion of high-quality protein, preferably with naturally occurring fat

- Choose from organic grass-fed meat, organic free-range poultry (skin on), organic free-range eggs and wild-caught fish.
- If you are vegetarian or vegan, choose a variety of organic legumes (ideally soaked before cooking, see page 230), nuts and seeds.
- Use healthy fats for cooking, and flavour with fresh herbs and spices for concentrated nutrition.

Include a side portion of starchy carbohydrate

- About ½ cup or 2–3 tablespoons.
- Choose from root vegetables, gluten-free wholegrains, pseudo grains or legumes (note: if you are vegan, include legumes as your protein source and choose either root vegetables, wholegrains or pseudo grains as your starchy carbohydrate).
- Choose gluten-free due to potential sensitivities and impact on gut health (see Start with your gut on page 17).
- Ideally soak legumes before cooking to improve digestibility (page 230).
- Cook with healthy fats (extra virgin coconut oil, extra virgin olive oil, virgin avocado oil, butter or ghee).

Dollop, drizzle or scatter with healthy fats

- Cook with healthy fats and use healthy fats for additional flavour.
- Aim for 1–2 tablespoons of healthy fat with each meal. This could include cooking with healthy fats or garnishing your meal with a drizzle of extra virgin olive oil, dressing (pages 204–207), nuts, seeds, olives, yoghurt or avocado.

Use concentrated nutrients liberally in cooking

- Cook with fresh herbs, organic spices and sea vegetables – they are both your nutrient and flavour allies. Not only do they make food taste great, herbs and spices also contain some of the highest concentrations of beneficial phytochemicals of any plant food.
- Some of my favourites are basil, cayenne, cinnamon, coriander, dulse, ginger, parsley, rosemary, turmeric and wakame.

Include two portions of unprocessed whole fruit daily (optional)

- 1 cup = 1 portion.
- Vary your intake through the six colours of the rainbow.
- Focus on the lower-sugar fruits such as berries. As well as being lower in sugar than other fruits, berries are especially high in antioxidants and fibre. Try adding berries to salads, granola (pages 140–141) or oats, or enjoy for dessert.

Berries are an ideal low-sugar fruit.

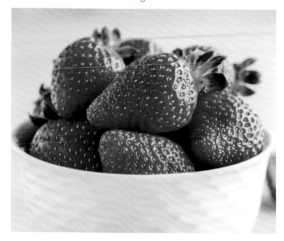

The Fertility Kitchen super foods

Eggs

Eggs are a rich source of complete protein, healthy fats and cholesterol. The yolks contain an abundance of important fertility nutrients and are the richest source of choline for many (the other richest source is liver, see below). If you're not sensitive to eggs, then aim to include two each day. If you're sensitive or allergic to eggs, or you simply don't like them, then it's important to focus on eating liver regularly and/or look at supplementing choline (pages 80–81). I've included plenty of recipes to help you eat more eggs (pages 126–130).

Leafy green vegetables

Green vegetables are especially beneficial for fertility because they are crammed with essential nutrients such as calcium, folate, iron and vitamin K1, as well as fibre. They also contain carotenoids, which are particularly concentrated in the ovaries where they protect against oxidative stress. Choose from chard (all varieties), collard greens, kale, rocket, spinach and watercress, and eat a variety. Aim to eat one portion (1 cup measure, tightly packed) with every meal. If it seems strange to eat greens at breakfast, add them to a smoothie (try The fresh green on page 138) or serve with eggs (page 129).

Liver

Liver scores highly in the fertility nutrition stakes; gram for gram, it contains more nutrients than any other food. It contains significant amounts of vital fertility nutrients, including vitamins A, B6 and B12, choline, copper, folate, iron, vitamin K2, selenium and zinc. If you haven't eaten liver before, start including it once a week and choose organic chicken liver, which has the mildest flavour. Hide small amounts in your favourite recipes by puréeing it or freezing,

Aim to include 2 eggs and 3 portions of leafy greens every day.

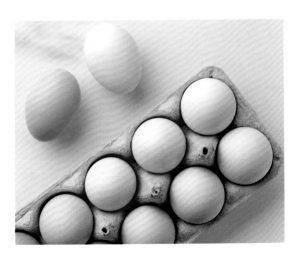

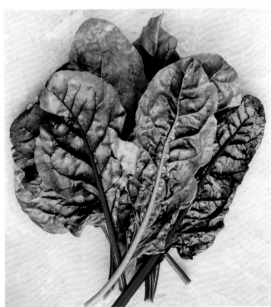

grating and adding it to the pot for the last minute or two of cooking time. Liver is suited to recipes like Bolognese, burgers, chilli and curries. Try my hidden liver recipes (pages 168 and 178).

Oily fish

Cold-water oily (fatty) fish is the richest dietary source of the essential omega-3 fat DHA. DHA is vital for foetal brain development, as well as lowering inflammation. Oily fish ticks a lot of important fertility nutrient boxes, including vitamin B12, choline, iodine, iron, selenium and zinc. Choose fish species with high levels of DHA and low levels of heavy metals (such as mercury) and contaminants. Good choices include Atlantic mackerel, herring, rainbow trout,

sardines and wild Alaskan or sockeye salmon. Include oily fish in your fertility diet two to three times per week and mix things up by trying different varieties. I've included plenty of recipes to help you achieve this. Try my Thai salmon cakes (page 151), Tandoori salmon skewers (page 163), Red miso, pak choi and crispy glazed salmon (page 148) or Mackerel with aubergine and cavolo nero (page 164).

Bone broth, meat on-the-bone and slow-cooked meat

Homemade bone broth (stock) offers a source of nutrients that can otherwise be lacking in our diets. The bones, skin and connective tissue are rich in protein, gelatine, collagen, glycine and minerals. Bones contain more minerals per gram than any other body tissue and broth made from bones is full of these minerals as they leach into the liquid as it simmers. Collagen and gelatine are rich sources of glycine, which is essential to obtain from the diet during pregnancy. Glycine is a structural amino acid required for foetal DNA and collagen synthesis. The most reliable sources include bone broth, slow-cooked meat and skin-on, bone-in poultry. You can also add pure gelatine or collagen powders to other foods. Try making a nourishing stock (pages 152–153), which you can use to make soups, Boosted broth for a daily tonic (page 153), Slow-cooked pulled pork (page 179), Lemon-and-herb-crusted roast chicken (page 172), Adaptogenic cinnamon-chai hot chocolate (page 227) or Gut lovin' gummies (pages 222–223).

Delicious salmon cakes (page 151) will help boost your intake of DHA.

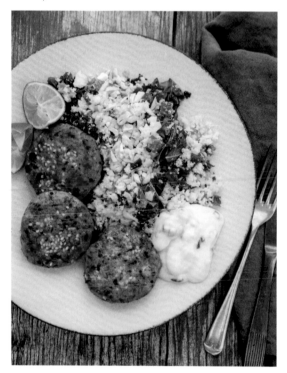

Five lunchbox ideas

Stuck for lunchbox ideas? I've got you covered with five nutritious suggestions to suit all dietary preferences. Adopt the 'cook once, eat twice' philosophy (make double at dinner) and you will always have something nutritious to box up for lunch the next day.

FISH

- 3 Thai salmon cakes (page 151) with 2 tbsp of Chilli lime dressing (page 204) and 1 serving of Thai-style egg-fried rice (page 195)
- 1 Power bar (pages 210–211)
- 60g (½ cup) fresh berries, 2 tablespoons of coconut yoghurt and 1 tablespoon of Granola (pages 140–141)

MEAT

- 1 beef burger (page 178) with 1 serving of Avocado and edamame smash (page 202) – squeeze with lemon juice to prevent it from turning brown
- 2 large handfuls of salad leaves of your choice and 1 tbsp Sauerkraut (page 191)
- Green apple with 1 tablespoon of almond butter

EGGS

- 2 Breakfast fritters (page 129) and 2 hard-boiled eggs
- 1 large handful each of watercress and rocket and 1 grated carrot with 2 tbsp of Yoghurt lemon dressing (page 204)

sprinkled with 2 tablespoons of nuts and seeds
- 2 Gut-lovin' gummies (pages 222–223)

VEGAN

- 3 Super-green falafels (page 142) with 2 tbsp homemade Hummus (pages 200–201) and 2 large handfuls of rocket or salad leaves of your choice
- 2 Almond and cinnamon fat bombs (page 215) – remember to pack a mini ice block to prevent them from melting!
- 60g (½ cup) fresh berries

PICK-AND-MIX IDEAS FOR MASON JARS

- Smoothie (pages 138–139) with 2 hard-boiled eggs on the side
- Veggie crisps (page 198) or Super-seedy crackers (page 146) with homemade Hummus (pages 200–201)
- Sticks of raw carrot, celery, pepper and cucumber with mixed nuts or Hummus (pages 200–201)
- Overnight oats (page 134) or Chia pudding (page 221)
- Fresh berries and coconut yoghurt with coconut flakes and cacao nibs, or Granola (pages 140–141)
- 1 slice of Seed and nut bread (page 136) spread with Hummus (pages 200–201), a hard-boiled egg and raw veg sticks
- Rainbow jar salad (page 154) with Green goddess dressing (page 205)

The Fertility Kitchen meal plan

Here's an example of a week of nutritious eating. Remember you can tailor your plan to incorporate your preferred mindful indulgences, consistent with the 90/10 approach (page 54). Stay hydrated by sipping on filtered water or healthy vitamin water (page 71) throughout the day.

	Day 1	Day 2	Day 3
On waking	Start-the-day tea (page 229)	Start-the-day tea (page 229)	Start-the-day tea (page 229)
Breakfast	Banoffee pecan granola (page 141) with coconut yoghurt and ½ cup fresh blueberries	Vanilla, coconut and passionfruit overnight oats (page 134)	The fresh green smoothie (page 138) and 1 slice of Seed and nut loaf (page 136) with scrambled egg
Lunch	Super-green falafels with cashew ginger courgette noodles (page 142)	Rainbow jar salad (page 154) and Green goddess dressing (page 205)	Glorious green soup with super-seedy crackers (page 146) 2 fat bombs (page 215)
Dinner	Tandoori salmon skewers with raita and onion salad (page 163)	Mediterranean roast veggie ragù (page 165) Coconut yoghurt with ½ cup fresh berries	Green dukkah-crusted cod with celeriac slaw (page 161)
Evening	Adaptogenic cinnamon-chai hot chocolate (page 227)	Anti-inflammatory golden milk (page 224)	Adaptogenic cinnamon-chai hot chocolate (page 227)

Day 4	Day 5	Day 6	Day 7
Start-the-day tea (page 229)	Start-the-day tea (page 229)	Start-the-day tea (page 229)	Start-the-day tea (page 229)
Fig, pistachio and honey oat bowl (page 133)	Banoffee pecan granola (page 141) with coconut yoghurt and ½ cup fresh blueberries	Apple pie pancakes (page 124) and a matcha latte (page 225)	Green shakshuka (page 130) and 1 slice of Seed and nut loaf (page 136)
Thai salmon cakes with chilli lime dressing (page 151) and Thai-style egg-fried rice (page 195)	Glorious green soup with super-seedy crackers (page 146) 2 fat bombs (page 215)	Red miso, pak choi and crispy glazed salmon (page 148)	Roasted butternut, tomato and puy lentil salad (page 158)
Easy weeknight curry (page 169) with Indian-style veggie rice (page 197)	Steak with chimichurri sauce (page 171) and sweet potato mash (page 194)	Green goddess cauliflower pizza (page 174) Chocolate hazelnut n'ice cream (page 217)	Lemon-and-herb-crusted roast chicken (page 172) Coconut yoghurt with ½ cup fresh berries
Anti-inflammatory golden milk (page 224)	Adaptogenic cinnamon-chai hot chocolate (page 227)	Anti-inflammatory golden milk (page 224)	Adaptogenic cinnamon-chai hot chocolate (page 227)

Smart supplementation

Supplements won't make up for a poor diet, however, they can help fill in nutrient gaps and imperfections in your diet and provide extra fertility support.

Supplement	Dosage
High-quality prenatal multivitamin	Daily, alongside a meal. Split the dose throughout the day to support absorption (e.g. half at breakfast and half at lunch).
Vitamin D3 (cholecalciferol)	4000 IU a day and possibly higher if you are deficient. Check how much is in your prenatal multivitamin and top up accordingly.
Choline (as choline bitartrate)	450–930 mg per day. Check how much is in your prenatal multivitamin and top up accordingly. 450mg is the current recommended daily amount for pregnant women, but studies have shown beneficial effects on foetal development and placental function at 930mg per day.
High-quality fish oil	Look for a supplement containing both DHA and EPA. A minimum of 300mg of DHA daily is required for pregnancy, although supplementation at much higher levels has been associated with positive effects on infant cognition.

Recommend brands	Notes
Seeking Health Optimal Prenatal, available as capsules, chewable or protein powder.	Avoid folic acid and instead choose a supplement with methylated B vitamins such as L-methylfolate (folate), methylcobalamin and/or adenosylcobalamin (vitamin B12) and pyridoxal-5-phosphate (vitamin B6).
Liquid drops in a carrier oil (vitamin D is fat-soluble) Thorne Research vitamin D (1000 IU per drop) or Seeking Health Optimal Vitamin D (2000 IU per drop).	Most prenatal vitamins don't provide enough. Deficiency is common, so it's important to test vitamin D levels (25 OH vitamin D blood test) via your GP or an online blood-testing service (see Resources on page 235) and increase the dose to address deficiency. Retest every 3 months.
Seeking Health Optimal PC Phospholipid Complex. 1–2 teaspoons per day – see notes.	How much you need depends on your diet and how much choline is in your prenatal multivitamin. If you regularly eat eggs and/or liver (the richest dietary sources of choline) and your prenatal provides 250mg, take 1 teaspoon. If your prenatal contains less than 250mg or you aren't eating choline-rich foods, then take 2 teaspoons.
Bare Biology Life and Soul Omega-3 liquid (contains Sicilian lemon oil so it doesn't taste fishy!). ½–1 teaspoon per day – see notes.	A fish oil supplement is especially important if you don't eat oily fish. If you consistently eat 2–3 portions weekly, then you can take ½ teaspoon. If you don't, take 1 teaspoon. Choose a supplement containing small varieties of fish (sardines or anchovies). It should be tested to be free of contaminants like heavy metals and PCBs.

The Fertility Kitchen pantry staples

I've compiled a list of pantry staples to help you find the more unusual ingredients called for in some of the recipes in this book. You can also find a list of my preferred suppliers on pages 233–234.

Almonds

Blanched
These almonds have had their skins removed. I find that blanched almonds work best for making almond milk as they produce a much creamier, smoother milk. You can blanch almonds yourself by soaking them in boiling water, allow to cool, then, using your fingers, slide the skins off.

Butter
Almond butter is made by grinding blanched almonds to a smooth, butter-like consistency. Roasted almond butter has a much richer flavour than an almond butter made from unroasted almonds. Check labels to ensure that the almond butter has no added sugar, salt, oils, preservatives or emulsifiers. The recipes in this book call for roasted blanched almond butter for its rich flavour.

Flaked
Flaked blanched almonds have their skins removed. They are a great addition to granola, porridge, soups, curries and salads.

Flour (ground almonds)
Blanched almonds are ground to a flour-like consistency. Almond meal is the same thing, although some almond meal is made from almonds with their skins on. As a flour replacement, blanched is preferable. Make your own by processing blanched almonds to a floury consistency in a food processor (125g almonds will yield 1 cup of almond flour). You can also buy extra-fine ground almond flour, which is ideal to use in smoothies or sauces where you want to avoid a grainy texture.

Milk
It's easy and more cost effective to make your own almond milk (page 137). You can control the creaminess of your milk by adjusting the amount of water you use. If you buy from a store, look for a milk that contains only almonds and water. Avoid additives such as oils and gums. My favourite store-bought brand is Plenish.

Artichokes
Artichokes are the immature flower bud of a thistle. The leaves (bracts) cover a fuzzy centre (choke), which sits on top of a meaty core. Artichokes have an earthy, herby flavour and make a great topping for pizzas (page 174) or a star ingredient in salads. Look for organic artichoke hearts or leaves in olive oil.

Baking powder
A raising agent used in baking to increase the volume and lighten the texture of baked goods. Most are gluten-free (check the label); buy certified gluten-free if gluten is an issue for you. Baking powder starts to lose its vigour when exposed to air, so you may wish to buy it in sachets, which is best if you use it infrequently. Look for an organic aluminium-free brand such as Bioreal, which you can purchase from Shipton Mill (online).

Banana chips

Banana chips have a crunchy and crispy texture; I use a small amount of these in granola. Be aware that they are not low in sugar, so use sparingly.

Buckwheat flour

Buckwheat is a fruit seed related to rhubarb and sorrel. Buckwheat flour is made by grinding whole buckwheat into a fine flour, while retaining nutritional goodness. Buckwheat is a great source of protein, iron and magnesium. Use this flour for baked goods such as pancakes and brownies.

Butter beans

Plump, cream-coloured legumes that have a soft, floury texture when cooked. Use them whole in salads, curries and ragù, or mashed or blitzed in soups. Some brands are now selling legumes in glass jars. A brand called Monjardin sell butter beans in

Candied beetroot (chioggia).

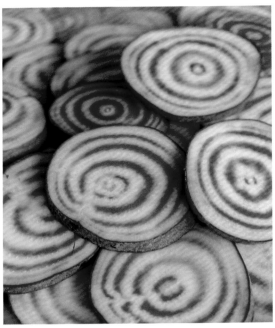

a 325g glass jar (available from Ocado), or you can buy them dry and soak them for enhanced digestibility (page 230).

Broccoli sprouts

Sprouts are baby plants, edible at just a few days old when they are at their peak of nutritional goodness. Broccoli sprouts are incredibly nutrient dense, containing up to 50 times the nutrients found in mature broccoli. Broccoli sprouts have a radish, peppery taste and are great sprinkled on salads, soups, curries or served with burgers. You can buy them from Abel & Cole.

Brown mustard seeds

Smaller and hotter than their relatives, yellow mustard seeds. I like to use these in Thai curries.

Candied beetroot (chioggia)

Beetroot, but prettier! I love candied beetroot for its vibrant pink. It's a great addition to salads for a pop of colour.

Capers

The cured bud of the caper bush, capers are dried in sea salt to preserve their distinct, aromatic and tangy flavour. Great in salsa verde and salad dressing, sprinkled into ragù or served alongside fish. My favourite brand is Moulins Mahjoub, available from Able & Cole.

Cashews

Cashew nuts (also known as kernels) are not actually nuts, but the seeds of the cashew tree. The seeds are encased in shells that adhere to the base of the cashew apple, the tree's fruit. Cashews have a lovely, smooth, creamy texture and are crisp to bite. Look for unroasted, organic cashews with no additives or preservatives. Cashews are great toasted and sprinkled onto stir-fries, curries and salads for an extra boost of protein and healthy fat.

Butter

Cashew butter is made by grinding cashews into a rich, butter-like consistency. Roasted cashew butter has a richer flavour than unroasted cashew butter. Check labels to ensure that the cashew butter has no added sugar, salt, oils, preservatives or emulsifiers. Add to smoothies and curries (especially Indian and Thai) or serve a dollop on top of overnight oats or porridge. The recipes in this book call for roasted cashew butter for its richer flavour.

Milk

Use whole cashews to make cashew milk (page 137). I find that cashews make the creamiest of all the nut milks and so I like to use it in hot drinks. If you buy from a store, look for a milk that contains only cashews and water. Avoid additives such as oils and gums. My favourite store-bought cashew milk brand is Plenish.

Cassava flour

Cassava flour can replace wheat flour in any recipe. It is made by grating and drying the fibrous cassava root, a starchy root vegetable. Use for Breakfast fritters (page 129).

Cavolo nero (Tuscan kale)

Also known as black kale, the leaves are very dark green, almost black, hence its name. You can use this in much the same way as kale.

Celeriac

A knobbly, odd-shaped root vegetable with a nutty, subtle, celery-like flavour. It's perfect in salads and slaws (page 161), or as an alternative to potato mash (page 194).

Chai spices

Available in a variety of blends. I like chai masala spices from Steenbergs (online). Use to make a warming tea or hot chocolate (page 227).

Chia seeds

Chia seeds are rich in omega-3, protein and a multitude of nutrients. Black and white chia seeds can be used interchangeably. White chia seeds are popular for baking and in chia pudding due to their neutral colour. Sprinkle on porridge, smoothies, salads and soups for an easy nutrient boost. Once opened, store the seeds in an airtight jar in the fridge to prevent rancidity.

Chickpeas

Chickpeas are a versatile legume that can be added to soups, stews, chillies and curries for an extra hit of protein and fibre. It's best to buy dried chickpeas and soak them before cooking to improve their digestibility (page 230). If you buy them ready-cooked, look for them in a glass jar, like the brand Biona Organic (available from Ocado and Amazon).

Chillies

Long red or green chillies tend to be mild and sweet, while small chillies are much hotter. Remove the seeds and membranes for a milder flavour.

Aleppo pepper

Sun-dried chilli flakes with a fruity flavour and medium heat.

Chipotle

Smoke-dried jalapeño chillies.

Chipotle in adobo smoky paste

A smoky, tangy paste made with chipotle chillies and tomato. Mix with oil and garlic to make a marinade for meat, fish or vegetables. I like the Cool Chile Company brand, which uses minimal ingredients.

Flakes, dried

Dried chilli flakes have been chopped into little pieces. They are great for sprinkling on soups, stir-fries and chillies for a flavour hit. Find them in the spice section in the supermarket or online from Steenbergs (be aware their hot chilli flakes have a powerful kick!).

Powder

Made from finely ground dried chillies. This can pack quite a punch. If you don't like hot flavours, then opt for a mild chilli powder. I use organic chilli powder from Steenbergs.

Chinese cabbage

Also known as Napa cabbage, it has pale, tightly wrapped, succulent leaves with crisp broad white veins and a delicate flavour. Use it to make Kimchi (page 192). Find it in your local Asian supermarket. Substitute with pak choi if you can't find it.

Chocolate (cacao)

Cacao/cocoa powder

Powder made from roasted cocoa beans. Cacao and cocoa mean the same thing. Use

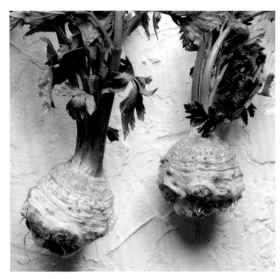

Celeriac.

for baking, to flavour oats, in smoothies and hot drinks.

Cacao nibs

Cocoa beans are cracked and winnowed (shells removed) leaving the raw nibs. I like to use these in place of chocolate chips, as cacao nibs are naturally sugar-free. Great for adding bitter crunch to oat bowls, overnight oats and power bars.

Ceremonial grade cacao

100% pure cacao made from high-quality Criollo cacao beans. I like the brand Forever Cacao.

Dark

The darker the chocolate, the less sugar it contains. My preference is 90 per cent cocoa solids. You can also get 100 per cent. Darker chocolate has a bitter, more intense flavour. Use it in brownies or dipped in almond butter for a sweet treat. Look for an organic dark chocolate made without soy lecithin, carrageenan or emulsifiers.

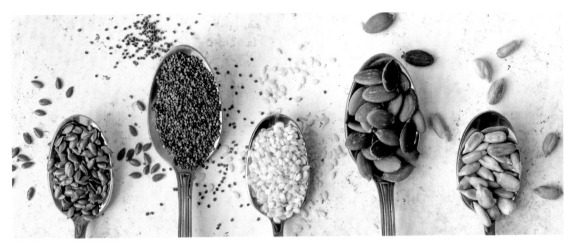

Flaxseeds, chia seeds, sesame seeds, pumpkin seeds, sunflower seeds.

Coconut

Aminos

A dark-coloured sauce, like tamari (gluten-free soy sauce). Coconut aminos is made from the sap of the coconut plant. It is both soy and gluten-free, so it works well if you are avoiding both. It is a little sweeter than tamari, so I like to add a small pinch of sea salt to aminos.

Chips (flakes)

Coconut chips are made from the pure white meat of coconuts, which is shredded and dehydrated at low temperatures. Coconut chips are available plain and toasted or you can buy plain and toast them in the oven yourself. Add to baking, granola, oats or curries. The recipes in this book call for 100 per cent coconut chips with no additives (such as sulphur) or sweeteners. I use the Coconut Merchant brand.

Cream

Coconut cream is a rich, thick cream made from coconut milk. It is the cream that rises to the top after the first pressing of coconut milk. You can buy this in glass jars from a brand called Nutural World. Add it to rice, curries, soups and hot drinks.

Desiccated

Desiccated coconut has a light, fragrant coconut flavour and is perfect for both savoury and sweet cooking. Use in baking, smoothies, sprinkled on oats or for adding a fresh taste of coconut to curry dishes. The recipes in this book call for 100 per cent desiccated coconut with no additives (such as sulphur) or sweeteners.

Milk

You can make your own coconut milk (page 137). Make it thinner by adding more water for a lighter milk (for use in overnight oats or pouring on granola) or make it thicker (for use in curries) by using less water. Otherwise, use tinned coconut milk in BPA-free cans for a thicker milk (look for coconut milk with no gums) and Plenish coconut milk for a lighter option.

Oil

The recipes in this book call for both extra virgin cold-pressed coconut oil and mild odourless coconut oil for use in cooking, baking, stir-frying, fat bombs, fudge and power bars. I like Biona Organic.

Water

The water from young, green coconuts, great for use in smoothies. I like the brand Rebel Kitchen.

Yoghurt

Coconut yoghurt is made from coconut milk and active probiotics. It is rich and creamy. I think COCOS make the best coconut yoghurt. The recipes in this book call for plain and vanilla. You can make your own vanilla flavour by adding a drop of pure vanilla extract to plain coconut yoghurt. Look for coconut yoghurt with minimal ingredients and no added sweeteners.

Dijon mustard

A traditional mustard of France, Dijon is pale yellow and creamier than yellow mustard, with less vinegar. Use in dressings. I like the brand Delouis, an organic Dijon mustard with minimal ingredients, available from Abel & Cole.

Dulse

Rich and smoky, purple dulse seaweed enhances recipes with its deep flavour. Sprinkle on salads, soups, stir-fries or omelettes. I like the brand Atlantic Kitchen.

Edamame

Edamame beans are whole, immature soybeans. Look for organic shelled edamame in the freezer section of supermarkets.

Eggs

The standard egg size used in this book is large (63–73g). Room temperature eggs are best for cooking. Use the freshest eggs possible for poached eggs (page 129).

Extracts

Almond, lemon, orange, peppermint and vanilla. For a pure taste, use a good-quality extract, not an essence or imitation flavour. Extracts are a great way to add flavour to a range of recipes, like granola (pages 140–141), Overnight oats (page 134), Fat bombs (page 215) and Power bars (pages 210–211). I like Steenbergs extracts. Available online.

Fennel seeds

Fennel seeds enhance both sweet and savoury foods with their mild aniseed flavour. The seeds range from green to yellow to brown.

Flaxseeds (linseeds)

Flaxseeds are also commonly known as linseeds and have a slightly nutty taste. Use in the Seed and nut gluten-free loaf (page 136). Store in a glass container in the fridge as flaxseeds are prone to rancidity.

Edamame.

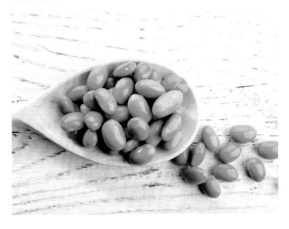

Milled sprouted

Sprouted flaxseeds have a superior nutrition profile. They are germinated, then slowly dried and cold milled. Use in smoothies, oats and baking. I like the brand Linwoods.

Garam masala

A traditional blend of Indian spices and one of the basic spice mixes of Indian cookery. Use in the Easy weeknight curry (page 169) and Curried cauliflower with almonds (page 190). My favourite blend is East End garam masala powder.

Garlic

Powder

A great way to add garlic flavour to food. Use it in dressings and sauces. I buy this from Steenbergs (online).

Salt

Enhance any meal by seasoning with garlic salt. I absolutely love to roast sweet potato with flavourless coconut oil and garlic salt – it's a simple side dish, but oh so good. My favourite brand is The Garlic Farm.

Black garlic

Black garlic is white garlic that has been heat-aged for many weeks. Unique in colour and flavour, it is sweet and syrupy, with hints of balsamic vinegar. Use in Apple and black garlic sauerkraut (page 191).

Hazelnuts

Butter

Hazelnut butter is made by grinding roasted hazelnuts into a rich, butter-like consistency. Check labels to ensure that the hazelnut butter has no added sugar, salt, oils, preservatives or emulsifiers. Serve a dollop of hazelnut butter on top of overnight oats or porridge. It pairs perfectly with chocolate.

Ground

Delicious, rich sweet hazelnuts ground down to a floury consistency. Stir into oat bowls, overnight oats or smoothies for extra nutrition. Can also be used as a flour replacement.

Milk

It's easy and more cost effective to make your own hazelnut milk (page 137). You can control the creaminess of your milk by adjusting the amount of water you use. If you buy from a store, look for a milk that contains only hazelnuts and water. Avoid additives such as oils and gums. My favourite store-bought brand is Plenish.

Hemp seeds (hemp hearts)

Hemp seeds have a delicious, slightly nutty flavour. Bake with them, sprinkle them, add them to smoothies or make your own homemade hemp milk. Hemp seeds are high in protein and a good source of dietary fibre, the essential fatty acids LA (omega-6) and ALA (omega-3), iron, magnesium, potassium and fibre. Find them online at Real Food Source or from supermarkets and health-food stores. Look for hulled or shelled hemp seeds, or hearts as whole hemp seeds have a hard shell and a slightly bitter flavour.

Honey

Raw

Raw honey is only strained before it is bottled so it retains most of the beneficial nutrients and antioxidants that it naturally contains.

Pak choi (bok choi)

Red chillies

Mooli (daikon)

Candied beetroot (chioggia)

Turmeric root

Manuka

Manuka honey has antibacterial, antiviral, anti-inflammatory and antioxidant benefits.

Horseradish

A pungent root vegetable, find it next to fresh root ginger in supermarkets. Adds heat to dips (page 202) and sauces and pairs perfectly with roast beef.

Lemongrass

A herb with a fresh, lemony aroma and a citrus flavour. Adds an instant zing to Thai curries.

Macadamia

Macadamia nuts have a delicious, buttery, slightly sweet taste and are crisp to bite.

Medjool dates.

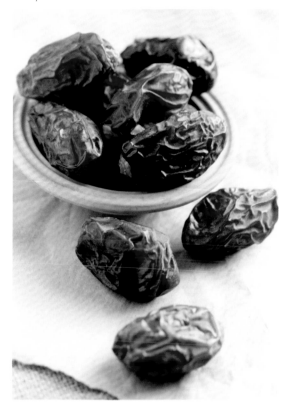

Sprinkle over salads, oat bowls and curries. Macadamias are a rich source of monounsaturated fats.

Butter

Made by roasting macadamias and then grinding them until a butter is formed. Check labels to ensure that the macadamia butter has no added sugar, salt, oils, preservatives or emulsifiers. Great for drizzling on oats, using in smoothies and for Salted macadamia and cashew butter fudge (page 213). I buy this online from Real Food Source.

Maca powder

Maca is a plant native to Peru. The edible part is the root, which is dried and made into a powder. Gelatinised maca has been lightly cooked, which improves digestibility. See Resources on page 235.

Matcha green tea powder

High-quality matcha should be bright, vibrant and rich in colour. The powder should be so finely milled that it wafts from the jar like smoke. My favourite is Lalani & Co Matcha Gold, a single origin matcha made from only one variety of tea. Most matcha is blended from various gardens. Look for an organic matcha so that it is free from pesticides. Matcha doesn't go 'off', but it will lose its nutritional value over time, so make sure you store it in the fridge after opening.

Medjool dates

Larger, darker and more caramel-like in taste than other dates such as Noor. They are soft and sticky. Use sparingly as they are a concentrated source of sugar. I use them in Power bars (pages 210–211).

Mexican chilli powder blend

A blend of chilli, cumin and paprika. Use to flavour Veggie rice (page 197) or as a dry rub for meat and fish. I buy this online from Steenbergs.

Miso paste

Miso is made from fermented soya beans, rice or barley, koji culture and sea salt. I prefer soya bean-only miso. Miso has a unique, salty flavour and aroma and an abundance of umami. White miso paste has a more delicate, sweeter flavour, while red miso is richer and more complex. The recipes in this book call for both white and red miso. I use Clearspring.

Mooli (daikon)

This is a form of giant radish with a mild flavour. It can be eaten raw or cooked. I use it in Kimchi (page 192). Find it in the fresh produce section of supermarkets or your local Asian supermarket.

Nutritional yeast

A species of yeast called *Saccharomyces cerevisiae* grown to be used as food. The yeast is inactive. Use in cooking for a cheesy flavour. Look for unfortified nutritional yeast flakes. Fortified nutritional yeast containing synthetic vitamins should be avoided.

Oats

The recipes in this book call for gluten-free rolled porridge oats. To make your own oat flour, whizz whole oats to a floury consistency in a blender.

Onion powder

A great way to add onion flavour to food. Use it in dressings (pages 204–207) and No-mato sauce (page 209).

Pak choi

A member of the cabbage family, pak choi (or bok choi) has crisp white stalks and tender green leaves. You can cook it like you would spinach. It's great in stir-fries or miso soup (page 148).

Passata rustica

An uncooked tomato purée, roughly strained of seeds and skins for a rich, chunky finish. I use this in cooking instead of tinned chopped tomatoes because it is available in glass jars. Use as a base for sauce (page 208), chilli (page 168), ragù (page 165) soup and curry (page 169).

Pecans

Delicious, buttery flavoured nuts. Use in granola, baking and sprinkle on oats.

Butter

Pecan butter is made by grinding pecans to a smooth, butter-like consistency. Check labels to ensure that the pecan butter has no added sugar, salt, oils, preservatives or emulsifiers. Use it in Granola (pages 140–141) or spread on a slice of Seed and nut gluten-free loaf (page 136). I buy pecan butter online from Nutural World.

Onion powder.

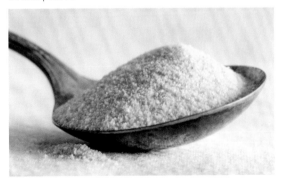

Pilau seasoning blend

Aromatic and spicy, this is a great blend to have on hand to season Veggie rice to go with curries (page 197). I buy this online from Steenbergs.

Pistachios

Pistachio kernels are rich, creamy and nutty in flavour. Buy de-shelled, roasted pistachios.

Butter

Made by grinding whole pistachios to a smooth butter. Use in Fat bombs (page 215). Check labels to ensure that the pistachio butter has no added sugar, salt, oils, preservatives or emulsifiers. I buy pistachio butter online from Real Food Source.

Psyllium husk powder

This a powder made from the husks of the *Plantago ovata* plant's seeds. I use this in my fibre-rich Seed and nut gluten-free loaf (page 136), you can also mix 1 tablespoon into Oat bowl recipes (pages 132–133) for extra fibre. Look for organic psyllium husk powder in health-food stores or online.

Pumpkin seeds

Flat oval-shaped green seeds. Use in granola, in baking and sprinkle on oats, soups and salads.

Puy lentils

Puy lentils have a delicate, slightly peppery flavour. See page 230 for soaking and cooking instructions.

Quinoa

A grain-like seed with a nutty flavour and light and fluffy texture. A great gluten-free alternative to couscous. See page 231 for soaking and cooking instructions. Use in Abundance bowls (pages 180–183)

Flakes

Quinoa flakes are simply quinoa seeds that have been rolled into flakes. Use them in baked goods such as my Seed and nut loaf (page 136) or in Power bars (pages 210–211) or Oat bowls (pages 132–133) in place of rolled oats. Find them in health-food shops and supermarkets. I buy mine online from Real Food Source.

Psyllium husk powder.

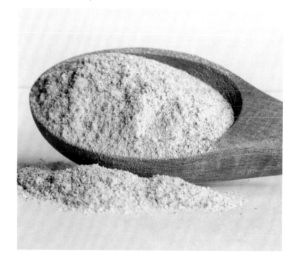

Quinoa.

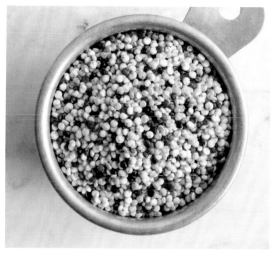

Sesame

Oil

A versatile oil with a delicate, nutty flavour. Look for cold-pressed oil and use in marinades and dressings. I like Mr Organic toasted sesame oil.

Seeds

These seeds have a nutty flavour. White sesame seeds are the most common variety and black (un-hulled) are popular in Asian cooking. You can find black sesame seeds in the spice section of the supermarket.

Tahini

A thick, smooth paste made from ground sesame seeds. It's available in jars in supermarkets and health-food shops, hulled (light) and un-hulled (dark). The recipes in this book call for light tahini for its slightly smoother texture and less bitter taste.

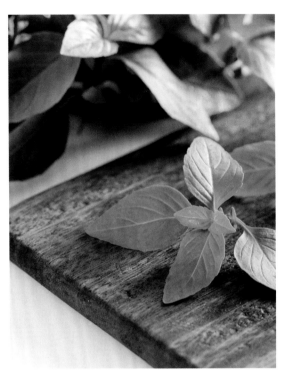

Thai basil leaves.

Smoked sriracha sauce

A type of sauce made from chillies. I like the brand Eaten Alive as they have sriracha made from smoked and fermented red pepper, chilli and onion. It's tangy and mild and can be added to dressing (page 207) for a spicy kick or used as a marinade.

Sunflower seeds

Small, grey kernels from the black and white seeds of sunflowers. Use in granola, power bars, in baking and sprinkle on oats, soups and salads.

Tamari

Tamari is a Japanese version of soy sauce but is gluten-free (check the label). I like the Clearspring brand. Use as a direct replacement for regular soy sauce.

Thai basil leaves

A type of basil with a sweet, anise-like scent and slight spicy flavour. Use in Thai curries and salads (page 157). You will find these in the fresh herbs section of the supermarket.

Thai spice seasoning

Available from Steenbergs (online). BART also do an aromatic Thai blend, which is readily available from supermarkets. Use in Thai-style egg-fried rice (page 195).

Turmeric

Fresh

A bright orange root found next to fresh ginger in the supermarket. Use in curries and teas.

Ground

An ochre-coloured, earthy-tasting spice. Use in curries and golden milk (page 224).

Vinegar

Apple cider (with the mother)

Organic unfiltered apple cider vinegar contains a cloudy substance called the 'mother'. It consists of strands of protein, enzymes and friendly bacteria. I like the brand RAW.

Mirin (Japanese rice wine)

Used to sweeten and give depth of flavour in Japanese cooking. I use Clearspring.

Sherry

Sherry vinegar has a non-astringent flavour that adds depth of flavour to cooking. Add a few drops to a finished dish as you would lemon juice or use it as the acid in Salsa verde (page 209) or chimichurri (page 171).

Wild blueberries

Frozen

Wild blueberries are smaller in size than regular blueberries. They have a more intense, sweet and tangy flavour. Wild blueberries contain twice as many antioxidants compared to regular blueberries and other berries, less sugar and more fibre. You will find these in the freezer aisle rather than fresh. Look for the brand Picard (available from Ocado).

Powder

Wild blueberry powder is a nutrient-dense powder that can be added to smoothies, oats, yoghurt or baking. One teaspoon of blueberry powder is equivalent to a handful

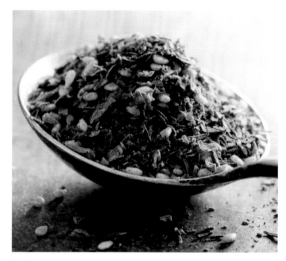

Za'atar.

of fresh berries. You can buy this online from Real Food Source.

Yellow split peas

Also known as yellow lentils and field peas. Soak this legume before cooking to improve digestibility, see instructions on page 230.

Za'atar

A nutty, earthy blend of dried herbs and spices. Za'atar is a versatile seasoning for hummus, vegetables, meat and fish. I love it with aubergine (page 184). Find it in the herbs and spices section in supermarkets or online at Steenbergs.

Equip yourself

The right tools make cooking easier and more fun. Here's my list of must-have kitchen tools that I can't be without. I recommend researching products to find brands that suit your needs.

- **Biodegradable parchment baking paper.** Look for the brand If You Care, which is plastic free and compostable.
- **Blender** (high powered). A Vitamix is the bee's knees of blenders and you have the option of buying a stainless-steel jug to replace the plastic one it comes with. A less expensive but still great option is the Magimix Le Blender, which comes with a glass jug.
- **Baking dishes and trays** in various sizes, including a loaf tin – I use ceramic and glass and line with plastic-free parchment paper.

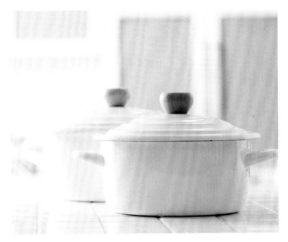
Cookware.

Kitchen staples.

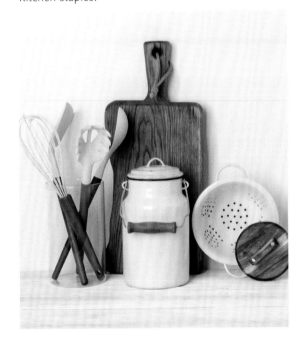

- **Box grater and microplane grater** for grating vegetables, zesting and finely grating fresh ginger and turmeric.
- **Colander** (metal or ceramic).
- **Cookware.** Cast-iron, enamelled cast-iron and high-quality stainless-steel pans and large wok. I use Le Creuset and Staub; they are an investment but will last a lifetime.
- **Food processor.** This is a handy kitchen tool for grating, mixing and puréeing ingredients. I use a Magimix.
- **Garlic crusher** for crushing garlic. My favourite brand is OXO.
- **Glass storage containers.** These are useful for food storage. Kilner and Weck sell a range of stackable glass containers, mason jars (including one for jar salads) and preserving jars for kimchi and sauerkraut. I recommend decanting nuts and seeds into an airtight glass jar and storing them in the fridge to preserve their nutrition.
- **Kitchen scales** for measuring ingredients that are hard to measure in cups.
- **Mandolin** for very fine slicing. I use one for Sweet potato crisps (page 198).

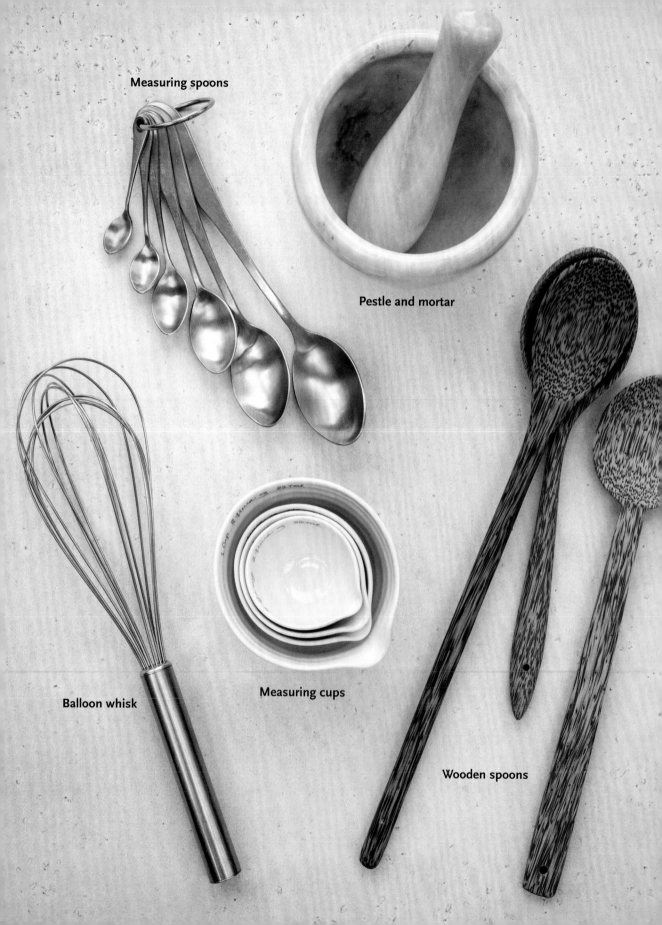

Measuring spoons

Pestle and mortar

Balloon whisk

Measuring cups

Wooden spoons

- **Measuring cups** (metal or ceramic). Sets of individual cups with handles come in 1-cup, ½-cup, ⅓-cup, ¼-cup and ⅛-cup measures (a 1-cup measure holds 250ml). They're brilliant for measuring ingredients like oats, ground nuts, seeds and raw cacao powder as they scoop so well. To measure properly with cups, take a big scoop and then use a knife to sweep over the top to make a level amount. Once you switch to cooking with cups, I guarantee you will wonder why you ever bothered to weigh anything! I encourage you to use cup measures for vegetable portions. Tightly pack leafy vegetables into a cup for one portion.
- **Measuring jugs** (glass) in two sizes.
- **Measuring spoons.** It's handy to know that 1 tablespoon is the equivalent of 3 teaspoons. Use level measures for baking powder, honey and extracts.
- **Mezzaluna.** I find this helpful for finely chopping herbs.
- **Mixing bowls** (glass or stainless steel. It's handy to have three in your collection – small, medium and large).
- **Oven thermometer** – this is a game changer for baking.
- **Palette knife.** Handy for releasing food from pans (e.g. power bars, fudge, brownies, frittata). I also use a palette knife to gently release cauliflower pizza bases from baking parchment.
- **Pestle and mortar (stone or wood).** Useful for crushing and mixing your own spice blends. I use a pestle and mortar to mix the rub for my Slow-cooked pulled pork (page 179).
- **Potato masher.** Use for Veggie mash (page 194).
- **Potato peeler and julienne peeler.** I have a potato peeler in two sizes (large is useful for peeling butternut squash; look for OXO large vegetable Y prep peeler). A julienne peeler will give you very thinly sliced vegetables; great for stir-fries and Rainbow jar salad (page 154).
- **Roasting tin.** I use Le Creuset 3-ply stainless steel.
- **Salad and herb spinner.** I wash all fresh vegetables (with filtered water) and dry them in a salad spinner before storing them in the fridge.
- **Serrated knife.** This will add texture to veggies and is great for making show-stopping salads.
- **Sharp knives** are essential. I use Kin Knives.
- **Sieves and sifters.** Always use a fine-mesh sieve for cacao powder.
- **Silicone moulds** for homemade gummies. Look on Amazon.
- **Skewers.** Metal or wooden for threading with meat or fish. If using wooden ones, soak them in cold water first so they don't burn.
- **Slow cooker** (you will need this for the Slow-cooked beef and black bean chilli on page 168).
- **Spatulas** in various sizes.
- **Spiraliser.** I use Kenwood electric.
- **Stick blender with mini chopper** and whisk. I use SMEG.
- **Temperature-controlled kettle** – for all that herbal tea! I use SMEG.
- **Tongs.** Useful for turning veggies and meat and tossing dressing through courgette noodles.
- **Whisks** – balloon whisk in 2 sizes (small and large) and a sauce whisk.
- **Wooden chopping boards.** These will help keep your knives sharper for longer.
- **Wooden spoons** in a variety of sizes.

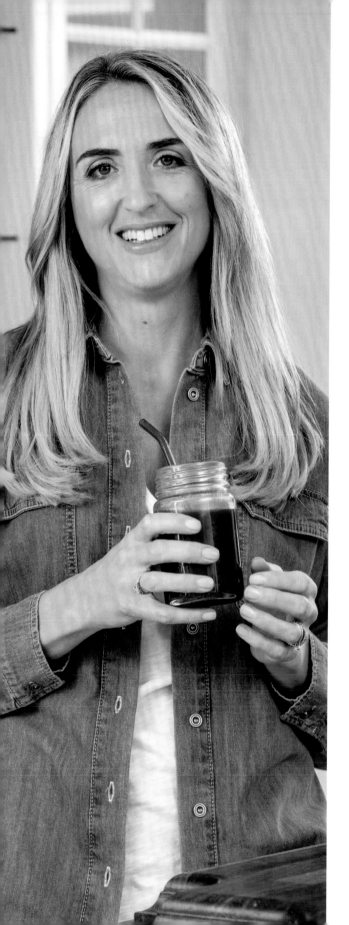

Life

Your health is made up of many small daily steps (stress, sleep, movement, environment and mindset) and these comprise the Life pillar.

Stress

Inside the stress response

When you encounter a stressor, your sympathetic nervous system stimulates the release of adrenaline and cortisol. These hormones prepare you for fight or flight by increasing blood flow to your heart, lungs, brain and muscles, raising blood sugar for a burst of energy, activating your immune system in case of injury or infection, and directing energy away from non-essential functions, like digestion and reproduction. When the 'threat' has passed, the parasympathetic nervous system takes over to counterbalance these responses and bring you back to neutral. In response to a temporary threat, this system works beautifully.

In the past, stress was short-lived. Once we got away from danger, these chemical messengers returned to normal. The problem today is that our bodies still have the same biological response, but we have more psychological stress in our lives. For many people, the stress response never switches off and this can affect every system in the body including hormones, digestion, immune system, metabolism, brain and mood. Chronic stress is a driving force behind many conditions, including fertility issues.

Stress, hormones and fertility

Stress directly affects the synchronicity of hormones and some of the problems that arise include:

Insulin resistance. Prolonged stress can lead to insulin resistance over time. Cortisol tells your liver to convert stored energy into glucose; simultaneously, insulin is released by your pancreas to regulate the newly elevated blood sugar. Consistently elevated blood-sugar and insulin levels can result in insulin resistance as cells stop listening to insulin's message. When the ovaries are exposed to consistently high insulin levels, they begin to alter their hormone production in favour of androgens (male hormones), interfering with ovulation and affecting fertility. Read more about blood sugar, insulin resistance and fertility on pages 22–26.

Low thyroid function. An elevated output of cortisol blocks the conversion of the thyroid pre-hormone T_4 to active T_3, instead promoting the conversion of T_4 to inactive T_3 (reverse T_3). This can be seen on blood tests with normal T_4 and low T_3. Read more about the thyroid-fertility connection on pages 31–35.

Low progesterone. Progesterone is vital for fertility. It rises following ovulation and creates an environment in your uterus to support a baby's growth by thickening the lining, reducing inflammation and changing secretions. Stress has an impact on sex hormones, and the interplay between progesterone and cortisol is a good example. Your body will always choose survival over reproduction. When the hypothalamus in your brain perceives stress, it signals to the pituitary gland to alter hormone production, reducing FSH and LH, which are both vital for a normal menstrual cycle, ovulation and progesterone production. In response to stress, the hypothalamus signalling the pituitary also signals the adrenals to increase cortisol production. Although it may appear that progesterone and cortisol have an inverse relationship, it is your brain that's in charge and its priority is your protection; having a baby during a famine doesn't make sense. However, your body will have the same response to modern stressors. Symptoms of low progesterone include infertility, short luteal phase, spotting and thin uterine lining.

Elevated prolactin. Prolactin is released in response to stress, and prolactin suppresses sex hormones, interfering with fertility. Read more about elevated prolactin and fertility on page 32.

Increased risk for autoimmunity. While immediate activation of your immune system can protect you from danger, chronic activation can lead to immune confusion, resulting in allergies, hives, eczema, frequent illness and autoimmunity. Read more about fertility and autoimmunity on page 15.

Time to unwind?

If you're regularly experiencing any of the following symptoms, then it's time to prioritise self-care:

- Feeling tired, but wired
- Anxiety, negativity and depression
- Feeling overwhelmed
- Irritability
- Energy slump in the afternoon
- Using caffeine to keep going
- Craving salty or sweet food

- Difficulty staying asleep
- Exhausted on waking
- Poor memory, concentration and motivation
- Weight gain around the waist
- Brain fog or difficulty concentrating
- Menstrual symptoms: severe PMS and symptoms of low progesterone: short luteal phase, spotting and thin lining

The stress-less solution

Practise gratitude. Gratitude is the practice of turning your attention to the goodness that is already in your life. I started doing this during IVF, when each night I wrote down three things I was grateful for. Even when I felt like I'd had a tough day, I began to recognise there were still many moments to appreciate. It doesn't have to be a big thing; it could be the sun shining, time spent chatting to a friend or a smile from a stranger. This simple practice helps shift the brain away from stressed and negative thinking to a more positive frame of mind. It's a powerful way to reframe your perspective on life. Research demonstrates that gratitude contributes to more positive emotions, greater enjoyment of happy experiences, increased ability to navigate difficult circumstances, better health and stronger relationships.

Keep a notebook on your bedside table. As part of your nightly routine, write down three things you are grateful for. The goal is not to pretend that everything is wonderful. Rather, it's to recognise that good exists alongside the challenges you face and to notice the ripple effect of this positive perspective.

Self-care is essential. Have you heard of the saying 'mother yourself before you mother another'? It's vital to embrace this concept to optimise your fertility. How can you expect to grow and nourish a baby if you don't nourish yourself? Taking time to rest and recuperate will do wonders for your wellbeing. It refreshes you and enables you to approach your relationships and health with more enthusiasm and energy. Build self-care practices into your week: acupuncture, massage or reflexology can be great ways to rest and reduce stress. If necessary, schedule non-negotiable self-care time in your diary.

Embrace stillness and be present. This is an ongoing practice, a moment-by-moment decision to be exactly where you are right now. You can choose to be mindful at any moment of your day by tuning into your senses. What can you see, feel, hear, taste and smell in this exact moment? When you are tapped into your senses you are mindful and present. With time, mindfulness helps you to develop awareness of your thoughts and beliefs such as those that lead to unhelpful actions, like reaching for sugar when stressed. Awareness is the first step to change; you might recognise that you tell yourself you *need* chocolate in response to a stressful situation. Mindfulness creates the space for you to look at that belief and ask yourself if it's true.

Disconnect to reconnect. Our phones have become our constant companions. The average adult checks their phone every 13 minutes, often at the expense of downtime and real-life connections with family and friends and our natural biorhythms. Constant access to social media and relentless streams of information (Dr Google anyone?!) displace the boundaries that keep us healthy and balanced. Exposure to the electromagnetic fields and blue light emitted from our devices adds further invisible disruption. Managing the time spent on your phone can help improve your state of mind and quality of life. Make the commitment to put your phone away during meals. Choose one day a week for a digital detox and switch off your phone for an entire day. Turn off all notifications and remove unnecessary apps. Take a break from social media, especially if you notice yourself feeling more stressed or anxious. Go out and leave your phone at home – it's not that scary, in fact it's quite freeing!

Meditate to help manage strong emotions. A regular meditation practice can help promote adaptability and resilience and reduce reactivity. Regular sitting for just 10 minutes daily can have a positive influence on your mental health, helping to reduce stress and anxiety. Grab yourself a meditation app like Headspace or Calm to help you master a daily practice.

Restorative yoga, also known as yin yoga, is where you position your body in supported postures and relax into them for up to 20 minutes. Your body opens gently, and you begin to destress as your parasympathetic nervous system takes over. Yin yoga is perfect for you if you're tired, exhausted, have trouble sleeping or difficulty in letting go of control. It can do

Try this

Your breath is an ally that can support you when you're feeling overwhelmed; it's your in-built calming system and pathway into the present.

The 4-7-8 breath
This is an easy and effective way to soothe your nervous system. Use this technique whenever you are struggling emotionally:

- With your mouth closed, breathe in through your nose for four counts, as if you are smelling flowers.
- Hold your breath for seven counts.
- Breathe out through your mouth for eight counts, as if you are blowing a candle to make it flicker but not go out.
- Repeat for ten rounds.

Belly breathing
This helps quiet the mind and bring you back into the present moment:

- Place one hand on your belly and the other on your chest.
- Take a slow, deep inhalation through your nose and draw your breath all the way into your belly. Notice your chest rise and your belly filling like a balloon.
- When you can take in no more air, exhale slowly through your nose until all the air is out of your lungs.
- Repeat for ten rounds and as you continue, see if you can extend your exhalation, aiming to breathe out for twice the count that you breathe in.

wonders for relaxing your mind and slowing down the never-ending thought stream.

Have sex. This is an important one when you're trying to conceive! Having sex with someone you love is an antidote to stress, improves sleep quality, reduces cortisol and boosts mood. Orgasms are good for your health and a great form of stress release. If your libido is waning then adaptogens, especially maca and rhodiola, may be helpful (pages 106–107).

The power of no. Advocate for yourself by setting limits to protect your wellbeing. Saying no is the ultimate act of self-care; it's like pulling a protective blanket around yourself. Listen to your body and recognise when it's sending you a desperate plea for

Connect with nature by meditating outside.

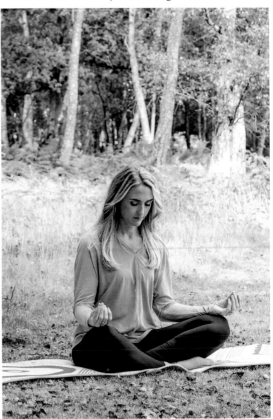

help. If you're feeling depleted or fatigued, you may have to decline a social invitation so that you can get an early night. If you're struggling to cope with infertility, you may need to say no to a baby shower or christening to protect your heart. It can feel challenging to say no and you might not be liked for it, but in the long run, those who count won't take it personally.

Prioritise sleep. Adequate, good-quality sleep is essential for helping you to manage stress. Lack of sleep and stress go hand in hand; sleep deprivation is associated with high cortisol levels. See pages 107–110 if sleep is an issue for you.

Drink herbal tea. Chamomile tea is well known for helping to evoke a sense of calm. Green tea may also be supportive because it contains L-theanine, a calming amino acid. Alternatively, make an Adaptogenic cinnamon-chai hot chocolate (page 227) part of your evening routine. It includes calming ashwagandha and nourishing maca to help you relax. Enjoy while reading a good book before bed.

Connect with nature. Being in nature is associated with improved psychological wellbeing. It has also been established that the more urbanised our environment, the worse our health. Have you noticed how you feel better after spending time in nature? It might be challenging or even impossible for you to spend time in nature every day, but at the very least you can spend some time outside. On your day off, commit to spending extended periods of time in nature.

Smart supplements for stress

Under the guidance of a nutritional therapist, consider the following supplements:

- **B VITAMIN COMPLEX. Pantothenic acid (B5)** is part of a B-vitamin complex and is essential for healthy adrenal function. It is thought to have the ability to reduce high cortisol production under stress. B vitamins help reduce inflammation and support liver detoxification. Although each B vitamin is chemically distinct, they work synergistically to support biochemical functions throughout your body, including healthy neurological function. Note that a B vitamin complex may turn your wee bright yellow – nothing to worry about, it's due to riboflavin (B2)!

- **VITAMIN C** is found abundantly in the adrenals and is depleted by stress. Sometimes vitamin C can cause digestive upset; a buffered vitamin C (where vitamin C is combined with buffering minerals) may help avoid this.

- **5-HTP** is a precursor to serotonin and may help if you're feeling anxious or sad. It may also help to restore motivation and support sleep by exerting a calming effect on the nervous system.

- **MAGNESIUM GLYCINATE** promotes relaxation and a sense of calm, and relieves anxiety and depression. My clients call this mineral magical due to its potent calming effects!

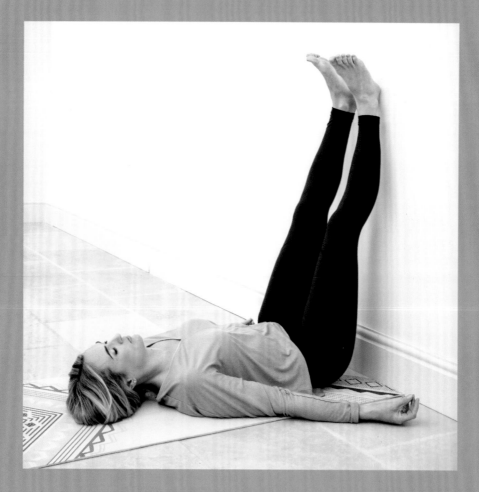

LEGS UP THE WALL POSE: A mood-altering pose believed to benefit the flow of life energy through the whole body.

Place a yoga mat against a wall. Sit on the mat, sideways to the wall about 15cm away, take your arms to the floor behind you and lean back. Swivel on your buttocks as you bring your legs up the wall. As your legs come up, rest your shoulders and head on the mat. Your chin, chest bone, pubic bone and big toes should be in a line, and you should feel supremely comfortable. Stay for at least 5 minutes and up to 15. To come out, bend your knees and roll out to the side. After several breaths, use your arms to push yourself up to sitting.

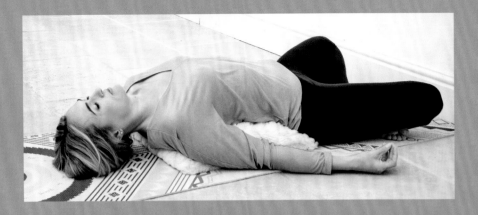

RECLINING CROSS-LEGGED POSE: Re-centre with this softly supported hip-opening pose.

Lie back onto your mat (you can use a bolster or pillow if you like), cross your legs and lay your arms out to the side, palms up, fingers softly curled. If you are not perfectly comfortable, adjust as required (you can use pillows or bolsters to support your knees). Cover with an eye pillow (if you like) and stay for 5–10 minutes. To come out of the pose, use your hand to bring one thigh up and slowly roll out to the side.

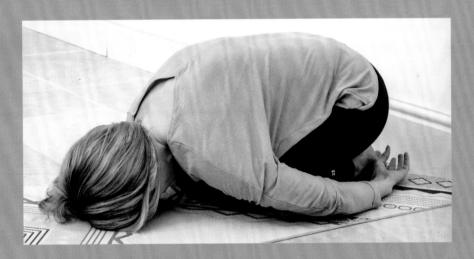

CHILD'S POSE: Enjoy turning your back on the world as you rest and travel inwards.

Kneel with your knees together. Sit back on your heels and fold forward to rest your forehead on the floor. Drape your arms beside your legs, palms up. Allow your shoulders to slouch happily. If your forehead doesn't touch the floor, try bringing your arms forward to make a little shelf for your forehead with one or two stacked fists.

Adaptogens for stress support

These are herbs that may help you adapt to stress and cope more easily with the demands of everyday life. Seek the guidance of a nutritional therapist or herbalist to help determine which adaptogen is right for you. My stress support favourites are:

- **Ashwagandha.** Known for its calming effects. Choose this if you're feeling 'tired but wired' or exhausted. It's also great for supporting sleep, especially if you find it difficult to drop off. Avoid if you're sensitive to nightshades.
- **Maca.** Considered 'the mother of all hormone nourishers' and thought to be very supportive to fertility. It is reported to improve libido and stamina, support hormone balance and reduce anxiety and depression. Try these recipes with added maca powder: Cinnamon omelettes (page 127), Salted almond smoothie (page 138) and Salted cashew and maca oats (page 133). Look for gelatinised maca that has

Get outside

- Drink your morning cup of tea or eat breakfast in the garden
- Eat your lunch outside
- Sit in the garden with a chamomile tea after work
- If you have a dog, walk it every day or borrow someone else's
- Connect to the earth by placing your bare feet on the ground or lying on the grass
- Practise yoga outside
- Join the National Trust and explore all it has to offer
- Take up gardening
- Organise a weekend hike or bike ride with friends
- Go camping (or glamping)
- Get some vitamin sea (visit the beach)
- Get involved in environmental activism, such as beach clean-ups
- Take part in outdoor adventures like paddle boarding or Go Ape.

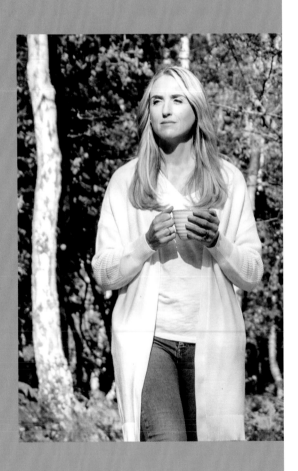

been gently heated to improve digestibility (see Resources on page 235).

- **Reishi mushroom.** Calms the nervous system and is useful in times of stress. Choose this if you feel chronically overwhelmed or anxious. You can get reishi in powder form, which can be added to hot drinks, smoothies, oat bowls or yoghurt, or in capsule form (more concentrated). See Resources, page 235.
- **Rhodiola.** Calming. Choose this if you struggle with anxiety, irritability or if you feel burned out. It is also thought to boost libido and support fertility.

You should notice positive changes in energy, sleep, mood or sense of wellbeing within a couple of weeks of taking adaptogens. If the benefits wane, take a short break and restart or try a different adaptogen. Discontinue when you suspect you are pregnant and before starting IVF. If you are taking prescription medication, check with your doctor before taking adaptogens.

Try this

Make a vanilla maca latte. Add 1 heaped teaspoon of maca powder and 1 teaspoon of pure vanilla extract to 250ml (1 cup) of oat milk. Whizz in a blender then transfer to a saucepan, place over a low heat and gently simmer for 5 minutes.

Sleep

Sleep is the ultimate pause you need at the end of the day to give your body a chance to rest and clean up. Your brain never stops working and its processes generate waste, which it gets rid of via the glymphatic system – your brain's waste-disposal system. Most glymphatic activities take place during sleep cycles and your brain's neurons dispose of most of their waste while you sleep. Studies suggest that sleep quality has an impact on your brain's ability to clear waste and toxins efficiently, and the deeper the sleep, the more efficient the waste removal.

Sleep stages explained

Sleep stages are important because they allow your brain and body to recuperate. There are four stages of sleep: three that form non-REM sleep and the final for rapid eye movement (REM). Stages one and two are lighter stages of sleep, and stage three is the deepest and most restorative. Stage four (REM) is essential to cognitive functions like memory, learning and creativity. You spend the most time in deep sleep during the first half of the night and as you continue sleeping, more time is spent in REM instead. Progressing smoothly multiple times through the sleep cycle is vital to high-quality rest.

The magic number

Not all sleep cycles are the same length, but on average they last 90 minutes each. Research suggests that five 90-minute sleep cycles are needed every night to reset your natural clock and cortisol rhythm, to ditch the chemical toxins that accumulate in your brain and body all day and for your brain to do the work of sorting and filing new information. The magic number is *at least* seven hours of good-quality sleep every night.

The sleep-wake cycle

Circadian rhythms are 24-hour cycles that are part of your body's internal clock, and the sleep-wake cycle is one of the most important. It is directly influenced by the environment, especially light. The circadian rhythm regulates the sleep-wake cycle and when properly aligned, supports consistent and restorative sleep, but when imbalanced can contribute to sleeping problems.

Melatonin regulates the circadian rhythm. It is extremely light sensitive; in response to morning light exposure your brain reduces melatonin secretion. Morning light also signals your brain to release cortisol, cortisol wakes you and should be at its peak in the morning. Melatonin and cortisol are in an opposite relationship; when melatonin is high, cortisol should be low and vice versa. When either of these gets out of balance, it affects your ability to sleep.

As well as regulating sleep, melatonin may influence fertility. Melatonin receptors are found on ovarian cells and the fluid in ovarian follicles contains high concentrations of melatonin and these levels rise with follicular growth. It may therefore play an important role in ovulation.

Are you sleep deprived?

If you experience any of the following symptoms, take the steps outlined below to help optimise your sleep:

- Stress and/or decreased tolerance for stress

- Blood-sugar dysregulation and insulin resistance (see page 23 for more on this)
- Increased hunger and appetite (lack of sleep triggers increased levels of ghrelin, your hunger hormone, and decreased levels of leptin, which curbs appetite)
- Weight gain and/or inability to lose weight (again due to sleep's relationship with ghrelin and leptin)
- Frequent illness (poor sleep suppresses immune function)
- Fertility-related symptoms include hormonal imbalance, irregular cycles, poor egg and sperm quality
- Poor sleep also increases the risk of chronic conditions like obesity, diabetes and heart disease.

The sleep solution

Doing all you can to support high-quality sleep is one of the most important ways to care for your body. Before you start taking steps to optimise sleep it can be useful to keep a sleep journal. Make a note of your bedtime, length of sleep, how long it took to fall asleep, sleep quality, restfulness, whether you woke in the night, what time you woke in the morning and how you felt on waking. Use this to track progress as you implement these recommendations.

Limit caffeine and alcohol. Even one cup of coffee or tea can potentially affect your sleep, and alcohol can interfere with the sleep stages. At the least, avoid caffeine during the afternoon. Read more about caffeine and alcohol on page 71.

Manage stress. Stress and sleep have a two-way relationship. Stress impairs sleep and can be a trigger for insomnia. See pages 99–107 for stress-busting strategies.

Balance blood sugar. Classic symptoms of blood-sugar imbalance include difficulty falling asleep and night waking. Addressing issues in this area may help support sleep (pages 22–26).

Ban blue light in the evenings from devices such as phones and tablets as it can trick your body into thinking it's daytime. Exposure to blue light suppresses the release of melatonin, delaying normal sleep onset and disrupting your circadian rhythm. Avoid or at least reduce blue light at night, including dimming artificial lights, especially in the hour before bedtime.

Prioritise sleep. Do whatever it takes to get to bed at a time that will enable you to sleep for seven to nine hours. Humans are the only species that deliberately deprive themselves of sleep without legitimate gain! It may seem like sacrificing sleep to watch another episode of a boxset is worth it, but remember that adequate sleep is vital to your mental health and ability to cope with stress. Next time you want to watch just one more episode ask yourself 'at what cost?'

Consistency is key. Maintain consistent sleep-wake cycles, even at the weekends. I know this is a hard one, but the body likes

Try this

If you really can't give up your devices before bedtime, buy a pair of blue-light-blocking glasses (see Resources on page 233). These specs filter out blue light with anti-glare lenses that shield your eyes, support normal melatonin production and improve sleep. Alternatively, install an app on your computer or smartphone that blocks blue light.

Smart supplements for sleep

Under the guidance of a nutritional therapist, consider the following supplements:

- **VITAMIN B6** can be helpful at bedtime if you are prone to night waking and morning fatigue because it helps to rebalance overnight cortisol.
- **VITAMIN B12** improves quality of sleep as it influences melatonin production, helping your body to regulate its circadian rhythm.
- **GABA** is an amino acid that supports sleep by promoting relaxation. It is thought to improve sleep quality and duration when combined with l-theanine.
- **L-THEANINE** may be supportive for sleep, because it helps promote relaxation.
- **MAGNESIUM GLYCINATE** supports sleep by promoting mental and muscular relaxation. Deficiency has been associated with insomnia. Magnesium may also help reduce restless legs and muscle cramps if this is an issue for you.
- **PHOSPHATIDYLSERINE** has been shown to reduce cortisol concentrations and help regulate the circadian rhythm of salivary cortisol and may positively regulate sleep quality.
- **REISHI** calms the nervous system, so is perfect to enjoy before bed to promote deep, relaxing sleep. Add 1 tablespoon of reishi powder to the Adaptogenic hot chocolate recipe on page 227.

regularity. It's a fallacy to think that you can forgo sleep during the week and make up for it at the weekend. It won't serve you. Get to bed by 10pm and get up by 7am everyday to support melatonin production.

Create an optimal sleep environment of complete darkness to support melatonin. Cover up LED lights on electronics (or remove them from your bedroom) and use black-out blinds or a sleep mask if your room isn't completely dark.

Establish a routine of sleep-provoking rituals to help prepare you for peaceful sleep:

- Epsom salts and lavender bath (page 101)
- Yin yoga (page 101)
- Meditation
- Curl up with a good book
- Turn off the lights early and light some candles
- Use a red lightbulb in your bedside light. Red is the wavelength that has the least impact on your body's circadian rhythm, so a red lightbulb is handy for reading before bed or if you need to get up in the night
- Keep a notebook by your bed to jot down any thoughts that pop into your head when you're trying to wind down
- Make your room a tranquil haven, free of clutter so that you feel calm and relaxed
- Drink a mug of chamomile tea or Adaptogenic cinnamon-chai hot chocolate (page 227)

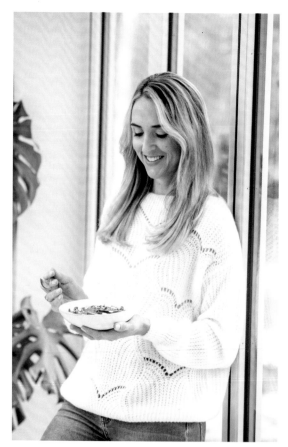

Find the brightest spot in your house to eat breakfast.

Early-morning light exposure, either by going outdoors or sitting near the window while eating your breakfast, helps trigger cortisol production and reset your cortisol awakening response.

Invest in a light therapy box for the winter months when the longer nights can disrupt bodily rhythms. Exposure to certain wavelengths of blue light that mimic the morning sky can have a strong effect on the night-time release of sleep-inducing hormones like melatonin. Use while eating breakfast or at your desk for 20 minutes first thing in the morning.

Movement

Physical inactivity and a sedentary lifestyle are associated with infertility. You may associate exercise with weight management, and while it can help with this, the benefits extend way beyond to encompass all aspects of health. Major benefits include reduced inflammation, improved insulin sensitivity and muscle gain. Both cardio and strength straining have been shown to improve glucose metabolism, which improves hormone balance and supports ovarian function. Regular movement also does wonders for your mood, and releases stress and tension from your body.

Move more

My movement principles are kind, gentle and moderate. Moving your body for 30–40 minutes a day in a way that you love is all you need to reap the rewards of exercise.

Make exercise non-negotiable. Create a routine that becomes a habit, like brushing your teeth. Plan and schedule exercise in your diary if you need to. The best time to exercise will be different for everyone – find what works for you and stick to it.

Be realistic. Progress over perfection applies to exercise too; it's much better to set realistic goals and be consistent than setting stretch goals that aren't sustainable. Take a step-by-step approach and eventually you'll be exercising most days and enjoying it.

Team up with a friend. As well as keeping each other accountable, exercising with a friend is more fun.

Mix it up. Your body (and mind) love variety. Consider a mix of yoga, Pilates, walking, swimming, biking and strength training. Variety is one of the best ways to get results.

Don't underestimate the power of restorative exercise. Yin yoga and walks in nature are great forms of stress relief (see pages 101 and 103).

Enjoy one or two rest days a week. Your body needs rest as much as movement, so don't feel guilty for taking a day off. The key is to be active, move your body every day and enjoy rest days when you need them. If you're having a stressful week, try yin yoga instead of pushing yourself to do an intense workout.

Are you over-exercising?

A key sign is irregular or absent periods. This can be caused by hypothalamic amenorrhea (HA), which is often driven by an energy deficit from undereating and over-exercising. If you are exercising intensely and experiencing menstrual irregularities, it may be that you are not eating enough to compensate for the exercise you are taking. When exercise is coupled with energy restriction (intentional or not), the hormones that regulate menstruation may be suppressed. There are other reasons for absent or irregular periods, such as PCOS, but over-exercising is a consideration if this applies to you.

Should you eat before a workout?

Exercise on an empty stomach; your body will use stored glycogen as a fuel source. After your workout, aim to eat a protein-rich meal within 30 minutes to replenish energy stores and repair muscles.

Solutions for sedentary living

Bringing movement into your day can be challenging, especially if you have a sedentary job. But, did you know that a sedentary lifestyle is now thought to be as bad for our health as smoking?! Sitting as a daily activity is not good for you, so get up!

Tips to bring movement into your day

- Park further away from your office, or if you're working from home, go for a quick walk around the block before you start work
- If possible, walk or cycle to your place of work instead of taking public transport or driving
- Take the stairs instead of the lift
- Use the furthest bathroom
- Take a break and walk outside for 5–10 minutes once an hour
- Do a quick set of jumping jacks, wall squats, push-ups, planks or yoga stretches whenever you can
- Swap your desk chair for an exercise ball or wobble stool
- Invest in an adjustable-height or sit-to-stand desk
- Bring movement into otherwise sedentary tasks by taking a walk while making your phone calls or have walking meetings
- Go for a lunchtime powerwalk
- Use a fitness tracker to track steps and aim for 10,000 a day. I love the Oura ring (see Resources on page 233).

Environment

A growing body of evidence links certain chemicals to fertility issues. Many other chemicals haven't been tested for safety in humans, so we know very little about their effect on fertility. It's therefore up to you to be discerning about what you put on, in and near your body. Keep the mantra 'progress over perfection' in mind as you read through this section. I know it can feel overwhelming to reduce your toxin exposure, but this is an area that can be fine-tuned over time.

Endocrine disruptors

Endocrine disruptors appear to be the worst offenders in relation to fertility. The endocrine system is made up of several glands that produce hormones. Endocrine disruptors are chemicals that imitate or partly imitate our natural hormones and are found in human tissue in much higher concentrations than the hormones our bodies make. They can overstimulate, block or disrupt our hormones' natural actions. Endocrine disruptors affect multiple systems in the body and have been found to contribute to both male and female infertility, miscarriage, endometriosis, PCOS and thyroid dysfunction. The table opposite gives an overview of the major players to look out for and avoid (this list is by no means exhaustive):

Endocrine disrupter	Where it's found	Potential fertility implications
Bisphenol-A (BPA)	Plastics in food/drink containers, coating in tinned food, plastic wrap, drinking straws, receipts and tickets	• Interfere with the activity of oestrogen, testosterone and thyroid hormones • Associated with poor egg quality and IVF outcome and miscarriage
Phthalates (plasticiser compounds used to extend the life of fragrances and to make certain plastics bendy)	Personal care products as 'fragrance' or 'parfum', air fresheners, synthetically fragranced products, scented candles, household furnishings, PVC flooring, food packaging (plastic wrap and freezer bags), nail polish	• May negatively affect sperm quality; linked to low sperm count and abnormal morphology • Associated with changes in male babies' testes and penis sizes • Associated with poor egg quality and impaired IVF outcome • May negatively affect follicular development and function, disrupt hormones and cause oxidative stress • Linked with miscarriage
Parabens	Personal-care products	• May interfere with male fertility; linked to low testosterone levels, abnormal morphology and poor motility • Associated with diminished ovarian reserve
Perfluorinated compounds	Non-stick cookware	• Linked to lowered testosterone levels and semen quality, abnormal morphology, female infertility and thyroid dysfunction
Triclosan	Antibacterial products, cleaning products, toothpaste	• Associated with decreased egg quality and poorer sperm quality • Linked to thyroid dysfunction

Minimising your exposure to endocrine disruptors

The top priority is to reduce plastics. This is an easy way to quickly reduce your exposure to bisphenols (BPA and the chemicals that are slowly replacing it: BPS and BPF) and phthalates. Heat, acid, UV light and contact with liquids are key factors that promote leaching of these chemicals from plastic.

- **Don't heat food in plastic containers – use ceramic or glass.**
- **Avoid washing plastic containers in hot water or the dishwasher and immediately replace plastic items that have been in contact with heat (preferably with glass containers).**
- **Use a glass or stainless-steel bottle/cup for water and hot drinks on the go.**
- **Say no to paper receipts – ask for digital – or wash your hands after handling.**
- **Replace plastic wrap (and aluminium foil) with beeswax wrap or vegan food wrap (see Resources on page 233).**
- **Replace baking paper and greaseproof paper with plastic-free parchment. I like the brand If You Care (Resources on page 233).**
- **Avoid canned foods (these are lined with bisphenols), ready meals, takeaways and other foods sold in plastic containers and bottles. Instead choose glass and opt for homemade meals, dressings (pages 204–207) and dips (pages 200–201).**
- **Store food in glass containers (see Resources on page 233).**

Why filter water?

Filter drinking water to reduce your exposure to fluoride (not currently applicable to all areas of the UK), chlorine, pesticide residues, bacteria and heavy metals. There is a plethora of water filters on the market. I like the Berkey water filters because they are made from stainless steel and filter out all the undesirables while retaining vital minerals.

Use glass jars and containers for food storage instead of plastic.

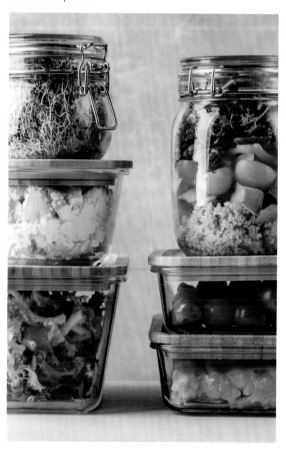

Detox your kitchen

Consider replacing the following items as and when your budget permits – don't stress about replacing everything at once.

Strive to replace	Safe to use	Suggested brands
Aluminium pans Non-stick pans	Cast-iron pans Ceramic and enamel pans Nickel-free stainless-steel saucepans	Le Creuset, Staub
Non-stick bakeware	Enamel bakeware Glass bakeware	Le Creuset Pyrex
Plastic bowls, including microwave-safe bowls, plastic jugs and colanders	Glass or stainless-steel mixing bowls and jugs, metal colander	Pyrex
Reusable plastic food storage containers	Glass storage containers and mason jars	IKEA, Kilner, Weck or reuse glass jam jars (if freezing leave 3cm at the top for expansion)
Plastic blender jug, especially if it has been used with hot liquids	Glass or stainless-steel blender jug	Vitamix (you can buy a separate stainless-steel jug) Magimix (comes with glass jug)
Plastic water filter jug	Stainless-steel or glass	Berkey

Detox your personal-care products

The main nasties in personal-care products include phthalates, parabens and triclosan, phenoxyethanol, resourcinol, benzophenone, polythene glycol, carbomer/polymers, butoxyethanol, ceteareth/cateareth-20 and microbeads (these are made of plastic).

Be wary of the words 'organic' and 'natural' on cosmetics labels – unless certified they don't mean anything, and the products can still contain undesirable ingredients.

- Stop using products with a strong scent; the worst offenders are perfume, hairspray and nail polish
- Simplify your skincare products – do you really need everything you are using?
- Replace items with cleaner alternatives as you use them up, like body lotion (highest priority), hair care, soap, deodorant, toothpaste, sun cream and makeup
- Look for paraben-, phthalate- and fragrance-free products (see Resources on page 233 for my favourite brands).
- Use the Environmental Working Group's (EWG) Skin Deep database or the Think Dirty app to check what's in your products.

Detox your cleaning products

The major nasties in cleaning products include phthalates, triclosan, glycol ethers (such as 2-butoxyethanol) and quaternary ammonium compounds.

- Prioritise removing bleach, air freshener and fabric softener – use natural wool dryer balls instead (see Resources on page 233)

Try this

Make this homemade all-purpose house cleaner, using only natural, easily available ingredients. If you think you will use this quickly you can use tap water, otherwise buy distilled water to prevent mould growth in the longer term.

2 litres water
125ml white vinegar
Juice of 1 lemon
50g baking soda
20 drops lavender essential oil, or tea tree oil for an antibacterial option

Place all the ingredients in a large jug, mix well and pour into a spray bottle.

- Remove all fake smells from your home (air fresheners, sprays, candles and plug-ins)
- Avoid optical brightener and dryer sheets
- Avoid antibacterial hand gels containing triclosan – you can replace these with alternatives such as Neal's Yard natural defence hand rub
- Replace detergent, spray cleaners, toilet cleaner, oven cleaner and soaps with cleaner alternatives as you run out
- Look for non-toxic alternatives free from the chemicals listed above (see Resources on page 233).

Mindset

The power of your mind is profound. How you talk to yourself matters because your thoughts impact your body, both physically and emotionally. A positive mindset supports healthy choices and enables you to sustain new habits in the long term.

Managing your mindset

Don't believe every thought. When a thought pops into your head, ask yourself 'Is that true?', they often aren't and don't serve us. Awareness is key and practising mindfulness helps create the awareness and space to challenge your thinking (page 101).

Be kind. Treat yourself like you would your best friend; listen to your thoughts without judgment and accept them. This doesn't leave space for negativity.

Don't compare yourself to others. Comparison puts us in a state of lack and can make us feel stuck, which can be heightened when we're navigating challenging times. Many of my clients tell me that they struggle when they see pregnancy and baby announcements. In this situation, setting boundaries with social media can be helpful. Unfollow any social media accounts or friends that make you feel anxious, sad or guilty, as well as anyone who promotes unrealistic ideas or who you compare yourself to. Stop comparison in its tracks by keeping focused on your own goals. Just because someone has something you want it doesn't mean that you can't or won't have it too. There is enough in life for everyone; focus on abundance.

Distance yourself from toxic relationships. If you dread being around someone, it's likely a toxic friendship that isn't serving you. Reflect on who is making you feel angry or upset when you see them. If they're a family member or someone you can't realistically cut out, consider gently putting up boundaries. Moderate the time you spend with them; see them less often or tell them you're focusing on yourself for a while.

Find your TTC sisters. I think everyone struggling with infertility has felt isolated and alone at some point. Audrey Hepburn once said, 'I am half agony, half hope' and to me this sums up the fertility journey perfectly. I think it's difficult for those not struggling with fertility issues to understand this, no matter how sensitive and empathetic they are. It is incredibly important to find others who understand the journey and won't offer (un)helpful advice, just a kind, listening ear. You can find a fertility support group through the charity Fertility Network UK (see Resources on page 235) or if there isn't a group in your local area, consider volunteering.

Connect with people who get it

- Find a community on Instagram. If you're not ready to go public with your journey, set up a dedicated anonymous fertility account.
- Join a Facebook group. There is a range of groups offering support for all aspects of trying to conceive, including The Fertility Kitchen Community, which you are more than welcome to join (see link on page 233).

Hateful to grateful. Your view of yourself and of the world is influenced by your belief system. If you have a victim mindset you may feel like everything is against you. This mentality is characterised by negative self-talk, such as 'Everything bad happens to me', 'It's not fair, when will it be my turn?', or 'I can't do anything about it, so why bother?'. Each new difficulty can reinforce these ideas and take a toll on emotional wellbeing, resulting in feelings of frustration and anger, hopelessness, hurt and resentment.

This mentality can be overcome with compassion and self-kindness. Positive mindset techniques are simple practices that can help shift your belief system. If the victim mindset resonates with you, find ways to make these practices part of your daily life:

Make time for the things you enjoy.

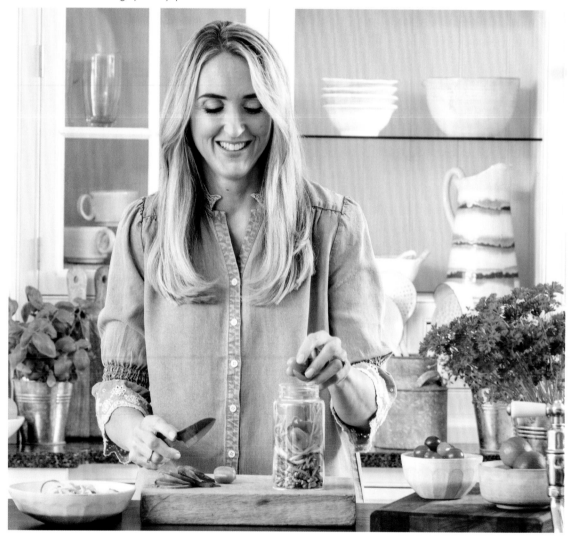

- Keep a gratitude journal (page 100).
- Practise affirmations. My favourite is, 'I am enough'. Choose the affirmations that resonate with you and repeat them often.
- Have fun. Make time every day to do something that makes you happy, e.g. reading, knitting, dancing, painting, gardening or cooking.
- Reframe your thinking. Reflect on negative moments and reframe them by thinking about what happened (as if you were an observer), what is the worst interpretation of your behaviour and then three reasons why that viewpoint isn't true. We all make mistakes and have moments when we're not the best versions of ourselves. Forgive yourself and move on.
- Forgive others. If a past situation or grudge is weighing you down, just let it go. Acknowledge and release it. I know it's easier said than done, but it will feel like a weight off your chest. Emotional heaviness can manifest physically, so forgiving a person or situation is freeing.

Let go of perfection. Ditch the assumption that healthy = doing everything perfectly. Perfect doesn't exist, and the pressure and anxiety that come with the idea of perfect set you up for failure. You can let go of perfection and still optimise your fertility. You don't have to do everything right all the time. I believe in a kind, balanced and flexible approach. Listen to your body, be guided by what it's telling you and do what feels good. When you feel good you'll have the energy to make healthy choices and take care of yourself.

Make health your focus and view it as a lifestyle. Optimal fertility is a side-effect of a healthy and happy body. View your health and wellness as a lifestyle to maintain forever.

Find your passion. When trying to conceive, and especially when navigating infertility, we may decline an adventure (like an exciting trip or activity) because we might be pregnant by then, or we stay in a job we hate because of the maternity benefits. It's so important to do what you love; plans can be changed. In the end, we have one life – don't put yours on hold.

Self-care checklist

Use this as a guide to help manage your mindset and make time for self-care everyday. You could make a note of these questions in your journal or write your own. Ask yourself:

- What is today's affirmation?
- What are my priorities today?
- What can wait?
- What one eating habit do I want to focus on?
- What self-care practices do I want to try (e.g. meditation, bath, breathing exercises, yoga, early night, digital detox)?
- When can I spend time outside today?
- How will I move my body today?
- How will I manage negative thoughts or feelings?
- What can I do to priortise sleep?
- What am I grateful for?

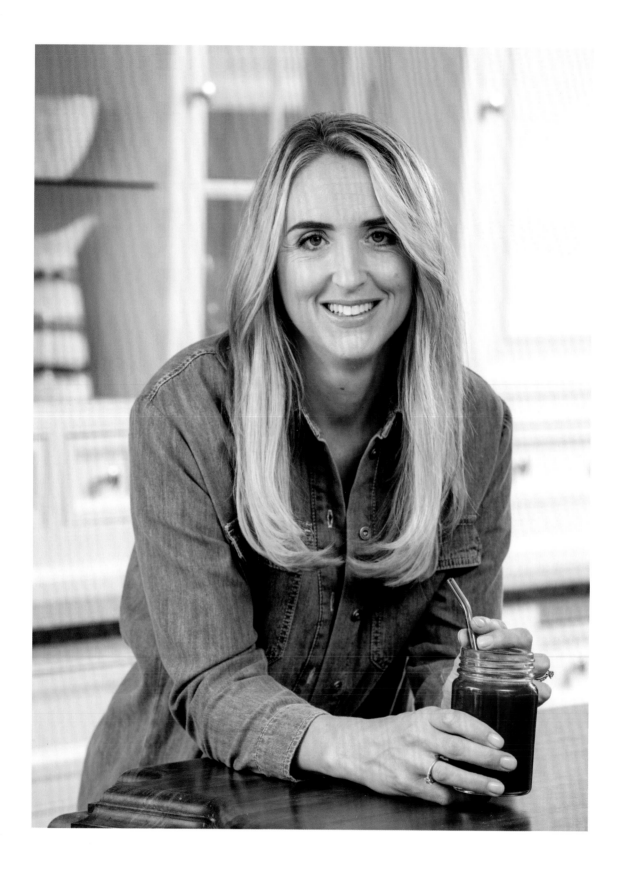

Final words

I wrote this book to inspire you to connect with, and listen to, your body and take control of your own health. The famous quote 'If you change nothing, nothing will change' is so apt; *you* hold the key to supporting your fertility. I hope this book provides the guidance and inspiration you need to advocate for yourself and that by making small but positive and consistent changes you will find a lifestyle that you can continue forever.

Remember, the goal is progress, not perfection. You can optimise your fertility by eating well most of the time, while also giving yourself the freedom to indulge, make imperfect choices, have a social life and simply enjoy life. To be healthy, we need to be flexible and committed to balance. If you can master this, it is truly liberating.

I believe in you. You've got this.

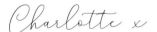

Keep in touch

I'd love to hear your story, so please stay in touch and let me know how you're getting on. Whether you want to share your pregnancy announcement or baby pictures, or if you're struggling with infertility, I'm here to support you. You're more than welcome to join my free community to share your fertility journey with me and other likeminded women. Look for The Fertility Kitchen Community on Facebook or follow along on social media. You can find me here:

Instagram: @thefertilitykitchen
Facebook: @thefertilitykitchen
Pinterest: @thefertilitykitchen

If you post a remake of one of my recipes or try any of my recommendations, remember to tag me @thefertilitykitchen and use the hashtags #thefertilitykitchen and #fertilityfoodlife so that I can see and share your creations and successes!

Finally, visit thefertilitykitchen.co.uk/book-bonuses to receive your free book downloads; these will be invaluable to help you get started. If you would like to find out how you can work with me, you can do that via my website too.

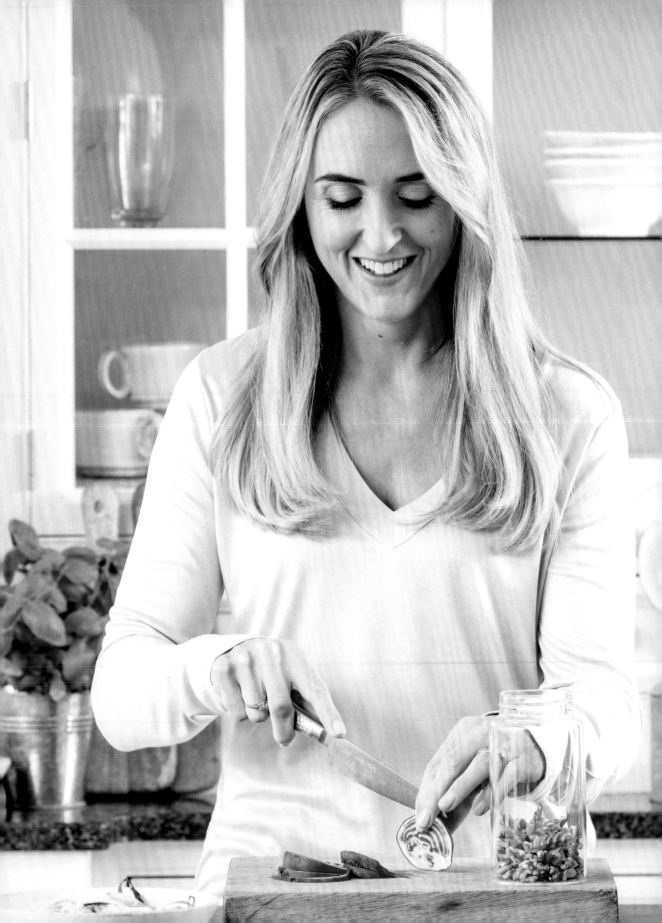

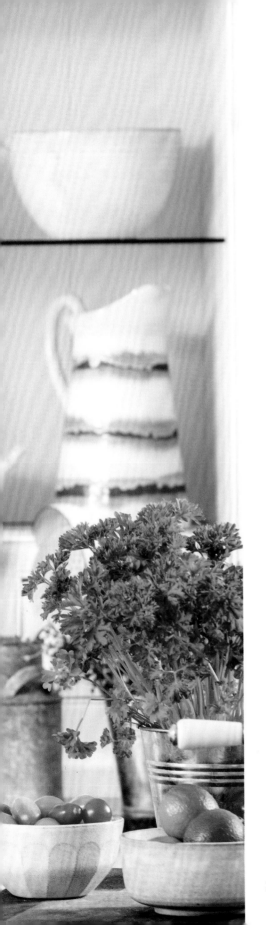

The Fertility Kitchen recipes

Apple pie pancakes

If you love pancakes, you'll flip over these easy, American-style fluffy pancakes. Stack them high and serve with fresh blackberries and a spoonful of coconut yoghurt. Enjoy occasionally for a special breakfast.

Makes 16 pancakes

120g (³/4 cup) gluten-free buckwheat flour
60g (¹/2 cup) gluten-free oat flour
2 tsp baking powder
2 tsp ground cinnamon, plus extra for dusting
2 medium bananas
1 large organic free-range egg

1 tsp pure vanilla extract
250ml (1 cup) gluten-free oat milk (to make your own, see page 137)
1 red apple, peeled, cored and diced
Flavourless coconut oil (or organic butter), to grease the pan
Vanilla coconut yoghurt and fresh blackberries, to serve

1. Place both the flours, the baking powder and cinnamon in a large bowl and mix to combine.

2. Place the bananas, egg, vanilla extract and oat milk in a blender and blend until smooth.

3. Make a well in the dry ingredients, pour in the banana mixture and whisk until smooth. Stir in the apple.

4. Heat a little of the oil in a frying pan over a medium heat. Cook heaped tablespoons of the batter for 2–3 minutes each side, or until golden (you can cook 3–4 pancakes at a time, just leave yourself enough space for flipping). Set aside and keep warm in a low oven. Repeat with the oil and remaining batter.

5. Stack the pancakes on serving plates and top with vanilla coconut yoghurt and fresh blackberries. Dust with cinnamon to serve.

Charlotte's notes

• Buckwheat flour adds a warm, nutty flavour to these pancakes.
• Make your own oat flour by whizzing oats to a powder in a high-speed blender.
• Leftover pancakes make great lunchbox fillers! Store in an airtight container in the fridge for up to two days or in the freezer for up to one month.

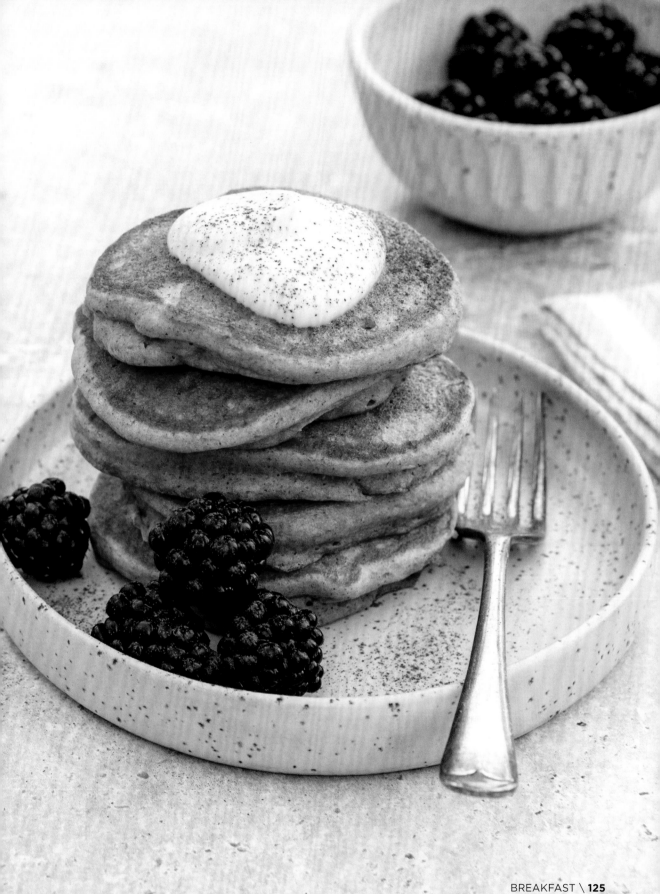

Turmeric-spiced frittata
with roasted tomatoes and yoghurt lemon dressing

Vibrant turmeric adds a splash of colour to this veg-packed frittata. This filling breakfast will keep you going all morning. It makes an equally perfect lunch or supper.

Serves 2

For the frittata

6 large organic free-range
   eggs
60ml (¼ cup) oat milk
   (to make your own,
   see page 137)
1 tsp ground turmeric
2 stalks of kale, stems
   removed and leaves roughly
   chopped
½ tsp sea salt

¼ tsp cracked black pepper
2 tsp olive oil
1 small onion, thinly sliced
6 tenderstem broccoli stems
   (about 100g), finely
   chopped
2 large handfuls of rocket,
   to serve
1 quantity of Yoghurt lemon
   dressing (page 204),
   to serve

For the roasted tomatoes

2 tbsp olive oil
2 tsp finely chopped basil
   leaves
1 garlic clove, crushed
200g (about 20) mixed
   cherry tomatoes on the
   vine
Sea salt and cracked black
   pepper

1. Preheat the oven to 180°C (350°F). Line a baking tray with plastic-free baking parchment.

2. First make the frittata, place the eggs, milk, turmeric, kale, salt and black pepper in a large bowl and whisk to combine.

3. Heat the oil in a medium heavy-based ovenproof frying pan over a medium–high heat. Add the onion and cook for 3 minutes, or until golden. Add the broccoli and cook for 2 minutes. Pour the egg mixture into the pan, stir to combine and cook for 2–3 minutes, or until the base is just set. Place the pan in the oven and cook for 12–15 minutes, or until golden and just set.

4. While the frittata is cooking, make the roasted tomatoes. Place the oil, basil and garlic in a small jug and whisk to combine. Spread the tomatoes evenly on the prepared tray, sprinkle with salt and black pepper and drizzle with the oil and herb mixture. Roast for 10 minutes, or until the tomatoes have softened. While the tomatoes are cooking, make the yoghurt lemon dressing.

5. Leave the frittata to cool slightly in the pan, then use a spatula to loosen the edges. Lift the frittata out of the pan and cut into triangles. Divide between serving plates and top with the rocket and roasted tomatoes. Drizzle with yoghurt lemon dressing to serve.

Cinnamon omelettes *with berries and cream*

A twist on a classic, this sweet omelette is quick and easy to make. Served with vanilla coconut cream, fresh berries and a dusting of cinnamon, it's sure to become a firm favourite.

Serves 2

For the omelettes
4 large organic free-range
    eggs
2 tsp pure vanilla extract
1 tsp honey
1 tbsp desiccated coconut
1 tsp ground cinnamon, sifted,
    plus extra for dusting
1 tsp gelatinised maca
    powder, sifted (optional)

¼ tsp ground nutmeg, sifted
2 tbsp coconut milk (to make
    your own, see page 137)
4 tsp extra virgin coconut oil
60g (½ cup) frozen mixed
    berries
Fresh mixed berries and
    desiccated coconut,
    to serve

For the vanilla coconut cream
2 tbsp coconut cream
1 tsp pure vanilla extract
1 tsp honey

1. Preheat the grill to medium. First, make the omelettes. Place the eggs, vanilla, honey, desiccated coconut, cinnamon, maca powder (if using), nutmeg and coconut milk in a medium bowl and whisk to combine.

2. Melt the oil in two mini heavy-based ovenproof frying pans over a medium heat (if you don't have mini frying pans, use a medium heavy-based ovenproof frying pan instead). Divide the egg mixture between the pans, sprinkle with the frozen berries and cook for 1–2 minutes, or until the bases are set.

3. Place under the grill and cook for 3–4 minutes, or until the omelettes are golden and the eggs are just set.

4. To make the vanilla coconut cream, place the coconut cream, vanilla extract and honey in a small bowl and whisk until smooth.

5. Leave the omelettes to cool slightly in the pan, then use a spatula to loosen the edges. Lift the omelettes out of the pan and serve on plates with a dollop of the vanilla coconut cream and a scattering of fresh berries. Sprinkle with desiccated coconut and dust with cinnamon to serve.

Charlotte's notes

• Gelatinised maca has been gently heated to improve its digestibility (see Resources on page 235).
• For a chocolate version, replace the ground cinnamon with 1 heaped teaspoon of cacao powder (sifted) and the desiccated coconut with cacao nibs.

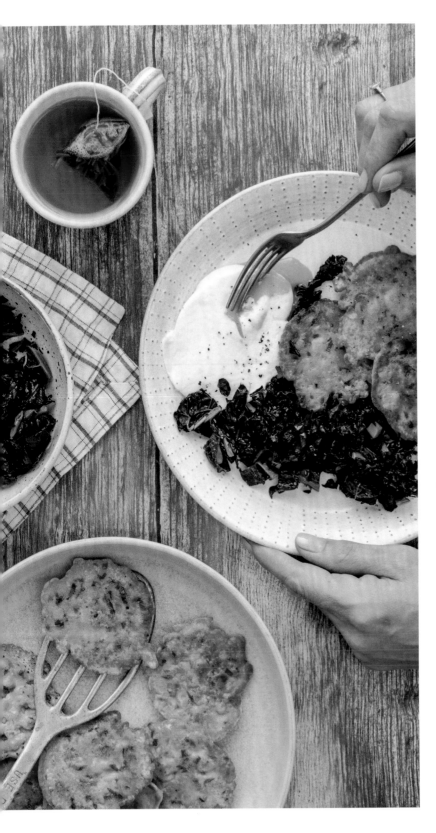

• Cassava flour (see Pantry staples on page 84) is a gluten-free flour very similar to wheat flour and has a mild, neutral flavour. If you can't find it, use gluten-free plain flour instead.

• Use the freshest eggs possible for perfect poached eggs. If you find it tricky to poach eggs, you can fry them instead.

• Leftover fritters make great lunchbox fillers. Store in an airtight container in the fridge for up to two days.

Breakfast fritters, *cavolo nero and poached eggs*

Mix up a pancake-style batter to make these delicious breakfast fritters, then serve with poached eggs and vibrant green cavolo nero for a healthy, protein-packed breakfast that will keep you satisfied until lunch.

Serves 2

For the fritter batter
60g (½ cup) cassava flour, sifted (see notes)
½ tsp baking powder
125ml (½ cup) oat milk (to make your own, see page 137)
1 tbsp lemon juice (about ½ lemon)
1 large organic free-range egg

Sea salt and cracked black pepper
120g (1 cup) frozen organic sweetcorn
1 small red chilli, deseeded and finely chopped
3 tbsp finely chopped flat-leaf parsley
Flavourless coconut oil, to grease the pan

For the cavolo nero
Olive oil, for frying
90g (3 cups, tightly packed) cavolo nero, roughly chopped
Pinch of sea salt
2 tsp lemon juice
Pinch of chilli flakes (optional)
2 large organic free-range eggs
Cracked black pepper

1. First, make the fritter batter. Place the cassava flour, baking powder, oat milk, lemon juice, egg, salt and black pepper in a medium bowl and whisk to combine. Fold in the sweetcorn, chilli and parsley. Set aside.

2. Next, prepare the cavolo nero. Heat 1 teaspoon of oil in a small frying pan and add the cavolo nero and salt. Stir-fry for 5–6 minutes, or until starting to wilt, then stir in the lemon juice and chilli flakes (if using).

3. Meanwhile, heat a little of the coconut oil in a frying pan over a medium heat. Cook heaped tablespoons of the batter for 2–3 minutes each side, or until golden (you can cook 3–4 fritters at a time, just leave yourself enough space for flipping). Set aside and keep warm in a low oven. Repeat with the remaining batter.

4. To poach the eggs, place a large frying pan over a low heat and pour in a kettle of just-boiled water. The water should be hot and steaming, but with no bubbles rising to the surface. One at a time, and keeping them well-spaced apart, crack in the eggs and poach for 3–4 minutes until the whites are set but the yolks are still soft. Lift out with a slotted spoon and drain on kitchen paper.

5. Divide the fritters between serving plates and top with the cavolo nero and poached eggs. Sprinkle with cracked black pepper to serve.

Green shakshuka

A twist on a traditional Middle Eastern dish, this green shakshuka makes the most of those all-important greens. Incredibly simple to make, shakshuka offers a quick way to get a very nutritious meal on the table super speedily at any time of day. This is my fave weekend breakfast.

Serves 2

1 tbsp olive oil
4 spring onions, trimmed and finely sliced
2 garlic cloves, crushed
1 bunch (25g) of coriander stalks, finely chopped
Pinch of sea salt
4 tbsp frozen pea and bean mix
2 baby courgettes, trimmed and sliced into ribbons
2 tenderstem broccoli stems, trimmed and sliced lengthways

3 tbsp Super-green walnut pesto (page 202)
80ml (⅓ cup) vegetable stock (to make your own, see page 152)
2–4 large organic free-range eggs

To serve
1 bunch (25g) coriander leaves, roughly chopped
2 large handfuls of rocket
Aleppo pepper, for sprinkling (see Pantry staples, page 85)

1. Heat the oil in a medium frying pan over a medium heat. Add the spring onions, garlic, coriander stalks and salt. Gently sauté for 2–3 minutes.

2. Add the peas and beans, courgettes, broccoli, super-green pesto and vegetable stock and stir until well combined. Use the back of a spoon to create 2–4 wells (depending on how many eggs you are using) in the mixture; crack an egg into each well and cover with a lid. Cook for 5–6 minutes, or until the eggs are done to your liking.

3. Divide between serving plates. Scatter with the coriander and rocket and sprinkle with Aleppo pepper to serve.

Charlotte's notes

• For a more traditional shakshuka, use Failproof tomato sauce (page 208) instead of Super-green walnut pesto.
• Try serving with a slice of Seed and nut loaf (page 136) to mop up the sauce.

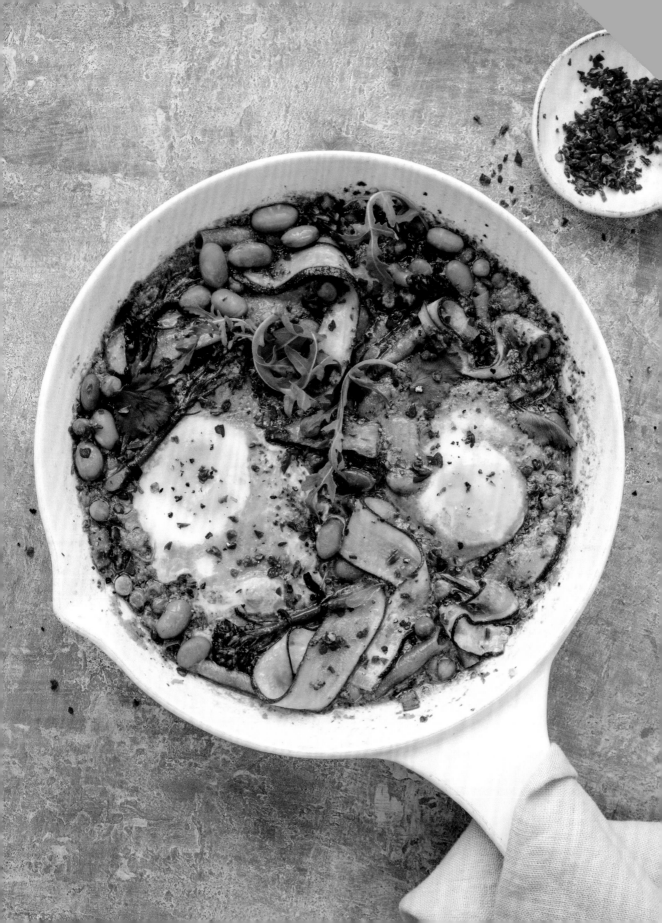

OAT BOWLS

Porridge is an everyday, feel-good breakfast. You can't beat a bowl of warming oats with delicious toppings to start a chilly morning.

The formula

Whole grain or pseudo-grain
30–45g (⅓–½ cup)

- Amaranth flakes
- Buckwheat flakes
- Gluten-free rolled oats
- Quinoa flakes

Liquid
160–250ml (⅔–1 cup)

- Filtered water
- Organic whole milk
- Plant milk (to make your own, see page 137)

Protein

- 1 large organic free-range egg, beaten
  +
- 1–2 tbsp ground nuts or seeds (almonds, Brazils, walnuts, hemp, pumpkin or sunflower seeds)

Toppings

- Coconut (flakes or desiccated)
- Chia jam
- Chopped or whole nuts
- Fresh fruit
- Granola (pages 140–141)
- ¼–½ tsp honey
- Nut butter
- Seeds
- Yoghurt

Flavourings
¼–½ tsp

- Extract (almond, lemon, orange, vanilla)
- Ground spices (cinnamon, nutmeg, ginger)
- Powders (cacao, maca, wild blueberry)
- Pinch of sea salt

Salted cashew and maca oats

Maca powder has a caramel taste and pairs beautifully with creamy cashews and a hint of salt.

Serves 1

30g (⅓ cup) gluten-free rolled oats
Small pinch of sea salt
160ml (⅔ cup) cashew milk, plus extra to
    serve (to make your own, see page 137)
1 tsp gelatinised maca powder, sifted
1 tsp pure vanilla extract
1 large organic free-range egg, beaten

To serve
1 tbsp smooth cashew butter
1 red apple, cored and thinly sliced
1 tbsp cashew nuts, lightly toasted and
    roughly chopped

1. Place the oats, salt, cashew milk, maca powder, vanilla and egg in a medium saucepan and whisk to combine.

2. Cook over a medium heat, stirring occasionally, for 3–4 minutes, or until the oats are thick and creamy.

3. Spoon the oats into a serving bowl and top with extra cashew milk and the cashew butter. Top with apple and sprinkle with cashew nuts to serve.

Fig, pistachio and honey oats

Easy to make and full of juicy fruit, this healthy breakfast will set you up for the day ahead. Porridge pairs perfectly with honey, fig and pistachio toppings.

Serves 1

30g (⅓ cup) gluten-free rolled oats
160ml (⅔ cup) almond milk, plus extra to
    serve (to make your own, see page 137)
1 tbsp ground almonds
1 fig, chopped
¼ tsp pure almond extract
1 large organic free-range egg, beaten

To serve
1 tbsp pistachio butter
1 fig, thinly sliced
1 tbsp chopped pistachios
½ tsp raw honey

1. Place the oats, almond milk, ground almonds, fig, almond extract and egg in a medium saucepan and whisk to combine.

2. Cook over a medium heat, stirring occasionally, for 3–4 minutes, or until the oats are thick and creamy.

3. Spoon into a serving bowl and top with extra almond milk, pistachio butter and sliced fig. Sprinkle with the chopped pistachios and drizzle with the honey to serve.

Vanilla, coconut and passionfruit overnight oats

A morning saviour! Get out the door fast with these make-ahead overnight oat and chia seed pots. Prepare them in a mason jar or jam jar for an easy grab-and-go breakfast.

Serves 2

2 tbsp white chia seeds
60g (2/3 cup) gluten-free rolled oats
2 tbsp desiccated coconut
2 tbsp hulled hemp seeds (see Pantry staples on page 88)
2 tsp pure vanilla extract
1/2–1 tsp raw honey (optional)
4 tbsp vanilla coconut yoghurt
160ml (2/3 cup) coconut milk (to make your own, see page 137)
Pulp of 1 passionfruit

Toppings, to serve
4 tbsp vanilla coconut yoghurt
Pulp of 1 passionfruit
2 tbsp toasted coconut flakes
Fresh raspberries

1. Place the chia seeds, oats, desiccated coconut, hemp seeds, vanilla, honey (if using), coconut yoghurt, coconut milk and passionfruit pulp in a medium bowl and mix until well combined. Divide between two jam jars, cover and refrigerate overnight.

2. In the morning, top with coconut yoghurt, passionfruit pulp, coconut flakes and a few fresh raspberries.

Charlotte's notes

Why not try these flavour variations?
• For lemon drizzle overnight oats, replace the desiccated coconut with ground almonds, the vanilla extract with 1 tablespoon of lemon juice and the zest of 1 unwaxed lemon and use coconut yoghurt and almond milk. Top with coconut yoghurt, flaked almonds and raspberries.
• For chocolate hazelnut overnight oats, replace the desiccated coconut with ground hazelnuts, add 3 teaspoons of sifted cacao powder and use hazelnut milk instead of coconut milk. Top with vanilla coconut yoghurt, hazelnut butter, chopped hazelnuts, strawberries and cacao nibs.

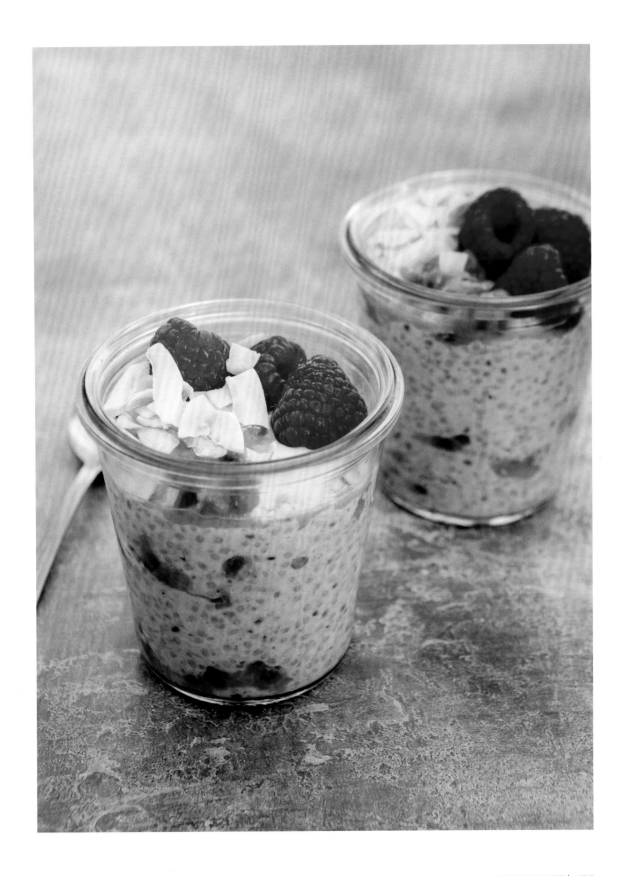

Seed and nut gluten-free loaf

This versatile loaf can be served topped with eggs and smashed avocado for breakfast, alongside soup for lunch or dipped into curry at dinner. I absolutely love it and make at least two loaves a week!

Makes 2lb loaf

85g (¾ cup) quinoa flakes (see notes)
85g (¾ cup) gluten-free rolled oats
85g (¾ cup) ground walnuts
2 tbsp white chia seeds
140g (1 cup) sunflower seeds
85g (½ cup) golden linseeds (flaxseeds)
3 tbsp psyllium husks (see Pantry staples on page 92)
1 tsp sea salt

4 tbsp extra virgin olive oil
375ml (1½ cup) filtered water
1 tbsp apple cider vinegar
1 tbsp honey

Serving suggestion
Sliced tomato
Avocado and edamame smash (page 202)

Charlotte's notes

• Quinoa flakes (see Pantry staples on page 92) provide a protein-rich addition to this loaf. You can use buckwheat flakes or extra gluten-free rolled oats instead if you can't find them.
• For a nut-free loaf, swap the ground walnuts for ground pumpkin or sunflower seeds, or a mixture of the two.

1. Grease and line a 21 x 11cm (900g/2lb) loaf tin with plastic-free baking parchment.

2. Place the quinoa flakes, oats, ground walnuts, chia and sunflower seeds, golden linseeds, psyllium husks and salt in a large bowl and mix to combine.

3. Place the oil, water, apple cider vinegar and honey in a large jug and whisk to combine. Pour into the dry ingredients and mix well to combine. Tip the mixture into the prepared tin. Refrigerate for 6 hours or overnight.

4. Preheat the oven to 150°C (300°F). Bake for 1–1.5 hours, or until golden brown and firm to the touch. Allow to cool in the tin completely before turning out and slicing to serve.

DIY plant milks

It's easy to make your own plant milk and much cheaper than store-bought versions. You can also be certain that it doesn't contain additives like oils or gums.

Makes 750ml–1 litre (3–4 cups)

Almond
150g (1 cup) blanched almonds
1.25–1.5 litres (5–6 cups) filtered water

Cashew
125g (1 cup) raw cashews
1.25–1.5 litres (5–6 cups) filtered water

Hazelnut
130g (1 cup) blanched hazelnuts
1.25–1.5 litres (5–6 cups) filtered water

Coconut
75g (1 cup) raw coconut chips (flakes)
1.25–1.5 litres (5–6 cups) filtered water

Oat
85g (1 cup) gluten-free rolled oats
1.25–1.5 litres (5–6 cups) filtered water

Type	Soaking time
Almonds, hazelnuts	Overnight
Cashews, coconut, oats	1–2 hours

1. Place the nuts, coconut or oats in a bowl and cover with 500ml (2 cups) of filtered water. Soak for 1–2 hours or overnight (refer to table above). Drain and rinse until the water runs clear.

2. Place the drained nuts, coconut or oats in a high-speed blender with 500ml (2 cups) of filtered water and blend until completely smooth.

3. Blend in another 250–500ml (1–2 cups) of filtered water, depending on how creamy you would like your milk to be (see notes), along with your chosen flavouring, if you are making a flavoured milk. If your blender hasn't completely broken down the nuts, strain through a fine-mesh strainer or cheese cloth. Store the milk in a sealed glass jug in the fridge for up to three days. Whisk or blend again before use.

Charlotte's notes

• Use less water for a creamier milk to use in hot drinks and smoothies, or more water for a thinner milk for pouring on granola or making oat bowls, pancakes or overnight oats.
• For a thicker coconut milk to use in curries, use only 400ml (1¾ cups) of water in total.

Smoothies

Smoothies offer a convenient grab-and-go breakfast for busy spring or summer mornings. I recommend eating a hard-boiled egg alongside your smoothie for an extra protein hit.

The fresh green

Show your liver some love with the freshest of green smoothies. There's more to smoothies than fruit – this green blend contains avocado, spinach, kale, parsley and mint for a super-healthy start to the day.

Serves 2

500ml (2 cups) coconut water
1 frozen avocado, thawed slightly
65g (½ cup) frozen pineapple chunks, thawed slightly
45g (1 cup, tightly packed) baby leaf spinach
1 stalk of kale
2 tbsp hemp seeds (see Pantry staples on page 88)
2 tbsp chopped flat-leaf parsley
2 tbsp chopped mint leaves
1 tsp grated ginger
Juice of 1 lime

Place the coconut water, avocado, pineapple, spinach, kale, hemp seeds, parsley, mint, ginger and lime juice in a blender and blend until smooth.

The salted almond

Whizz up a quick and filling salty-sweet almond butter smoothie. This creamy smoothie packs in plenty of nutritious ingredients, such as spinach, avocado and hemp seeds, with an optional spoonful of maca powder for a natural energy boost.

Serves 2

500ml (2 cups) almond milk (to make your own, see page 137)
½ frozen avocado, thawed slightly
½ frozen banana, thawed slightly
45g (1 cup, tightly packed) baby leaf spinach (optional, spinach will turn the smoothie slightly browner)
2 tbsp hemp seeds (see Pantry staples on page 88)
2 tbsp almond butter
1 tsp ground cinnamon
1 tsp gelatinised maca powder (optional – see Resources on page 235)
¼ tsp sea salt
1–1½ tsp honey (optional)

Place the almond milk, avocado, banana, spinach (if using), hemp seeds, almond butter, maca powder (if using) and salt in a blender and blend until smooth. Add 1–1½ teaspoons of honey to taste (if using) and blend again.

A berry good start

Antioxidant-rich wild blueberries give this smoothie its deep, purple colour. This is the original IVF protein smoothie that I drank every day during treatment. It's not the sweetest, but it's full of good things.

Serves 2

500ml (2 cups) cashew milk (to make your own, see page 137)

½ frozen avocado, thawed slightly

1 frozen banana, thawed slightly

45g (1 cup, tightly packed) baby leaf spinach

2 tbsp hulled hemp seeds (see Pantry staples on page 88)

1 tbsp ground flaxseeds

125g (1 cup) frozen wild blueberries

1 tsp wild blueberry powder (see Pantry staples on page 94)

2 servings collagen powder (see Resources on page 235)

2 tsp pure vanilla extract

Place the cashew milk, avocado, banana, spinach, hemp seeds, flaxseeds, blueberries, blueberry powder, collagen powder and vanilla extract in a blender and blend until smooth.

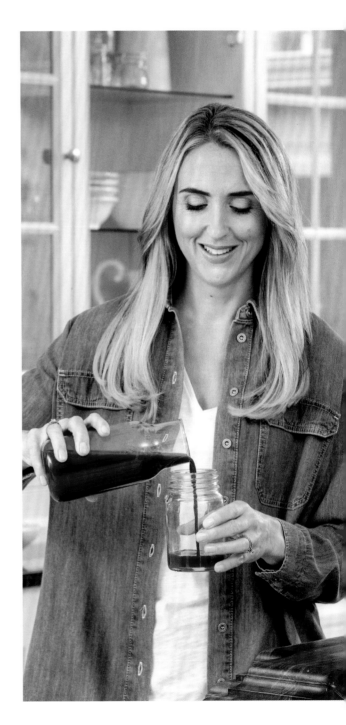

MASTER THE ART

GRANOLA

Make your own low-sugar granola packed with nuts and seeds for a nutrient- and fibre-rich breakfast. Serve with your milk of choice, yoghurt and fresh berries, or use as a topping for Oat bowls (pages 132–133) or Overnight oats (page 134). Granola will keep in an airtight glass container for up to four weeks.

The formula

Base ingredients

- 260g (2 cups) mixed nuts
- 75g (1 cup) coconut flakes
- 135g (1 cup) sunflower seeds
- 80g (½ cup) pumpkin seeds
- 45g (¼ cup) chia seeds
- ¼ tsp sea salt
  +
- 90–130g (1 cup) nuts of choice

Binding ingredients

- 50g (¼ cup) flavourless or extra virgin coconut oil
- 2 tbsp honey
  +
- 60g (¼ cup) nut butter of choice

Flavourings

To the base ingredients add any of the following according to your flavour preference:
- 2 tsp ground spices (cinnamon, nutmeg, ginger)
- ½ tsp–1 tbsp pure extract (almond, orange, peppermint, vanilla)
- 1–2 tbsp powder (cacao, blueberry, raspberry, strawberry)

Flavourings to stir through (optional)

- 30–60g (¼–½ cup) cacao nibs
- 25–50g (¼–½ cup) dried fruit (banana chips, chopped dates, goji berries, tart unsulphured cherries) – less is more as dried fruit is a concentrated source of sugar

Makes 800g (6 cups) / serves 8

Banoffee pecan

This is hands down one of my favourite granolas – a classic combination with a healthy twist.

To the base dry ingredients add
90g (1 cup) pecan halves
2 tsp ground cinnamon

To the binding ingredients add
60g (¼ cup) smooth pecan butter

To stir through the baked granola
50g (½ cup) banana chips, roughly chopped

Vanilla chocolate cashew

Chocoholic? You're in good company. Chocolatey and healthy, this is the perfect granola for chocolate lovers!

To the base dry ingredients add
125g (1 cup) cashew halves
2 tbsp raw cacao powder, sifted
1 tbsp pure vanilla extract

To the binding ingredients add
60g (¼ cup) smooth cashew butter

To stir through the baked granola
60g (½ cup) cacao nibs

Cherry almond

Is there any combination more delicious than cherry and almond? This granola combines both flavours for a protein-packed treat.

To the base dry ingredients add
90g (1 cup) blanched almond flakes
½ tsp pure almond extract

To the binding ingredients add
60g (¼ cup) smooth almond butter

To stir through the baked granola
50g (½ cup) unsweetened tart cherries (unsulphured)

1. Preheat the oven to 150°C (300°F). Line a baking tray with plastic-free baking parchment.

2. Place the nuts, coconut flakes, seeds, salt and flavourings in a large bowl and mix to combine.

3. Melt the oil, honey and nut butter in a small saucepan over a low heat, whisking for 3–4 minutes, or until smooth. Add to the dry ingredients and mix until the nuts and seeds are well coated.

4. Spread the mixture evenly on the prepared baking tray and bake, stirring occasionally, for 10–15 minutes, or until golden. Allow to cool completely, then stir through the banana chips, cacao nibs or tart cherries, depending on which flavour you are making.

5. Serve 100g (¾ cup) of granola in bowls with yoghurt and fresh berries.

Super-green falafels
with cashew ginger courgette noodles

Falafels make an easy, satisfying vegan lunch or delicious speedy supper. They pair perfectly with homemade Hummus (pages 200–201).

Makes 22 falafels

1 x 400g jar chickpeas, drained and rinsed thoroughly
2 garlic cloves, crushed
1 onion, finely chopped
125g (1 cup) frozen peas
4 tbsp ground flaxseeds
½ small head of broccoli (about 100g), roughly chopped

70g (2 cups, tightly packed) kale leaves, roughly chopped
1 bunch (25g) flat-leaf parsley
½ bunch (12g) mint leaves
2 tsp ground coriander
1 tsp ground cumin
Juice and zest of ½ lemon
½ tsp sea salt
¼ tsp cracked black pepper

Extra virgin olive oil, for brushing
Cashew ginger sauce (page 208, ½ quantity serves 2)
1 tsp olive oil per courgette
Courgette (1 per person), spiralised
Rocket leaves (large handful per person), to serve

1. Preheat oven to 180°C (350°F). Line a large baking tray with plastic-free baking parchment.

2. To make the falafels, place the chickpeas, garlic, onion, peas, flaxseeds, broccoli, kale, parsley, mint, ground coriander, ground cumin, lemon juice and zest, salt and cracked black pepper in a food processor and process until the mixture comes together.

3. Roll into 22 walnut-sized balls, place on the prepared tray and refrigerate for 30 minutes or overnight to firm up. Brush with oil and bake for 20 minutes.

4. Meanwhile, make the cashew ginger sauce and set aside. Heat the olive oil in a frying pan over a low heat. Add the courgette and cook for 1–2 minutes until warmed through. Drizzle with the cashew ginger sauce and toss to coat.

5. Divide the courgette noodles between serving bowls, add 3–4 falafels per person and scatter with rocket leaves to serve.

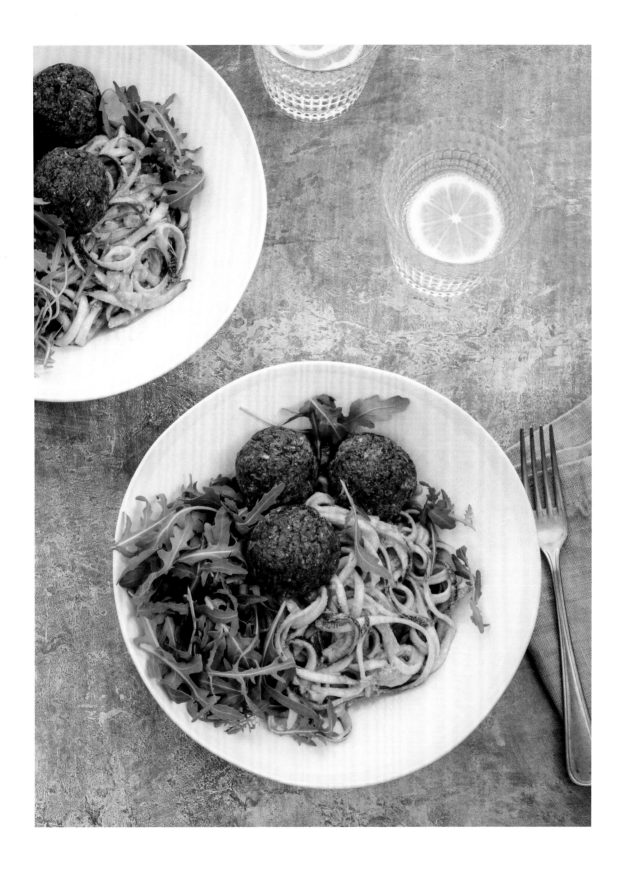

Creamy cauliflower soup *with salsa verde*

Cauliflower can be a neglected veggie, but it is one of my faves. It makes a delicious, delicately flavoured soup. The salsa verde, full of green goodness, brings a piquant quality to this velvety soup.

Serves 2

2 tsp Salsa verde (page 209)
1 tbsp extra virgin olive oil
1 small onion, chopped
1 garlic clove, sliced
1 small leek, trimmed and sliced
1 small cauliflower (about 300g), cut into
　florets

Sea salt and cracked black pepper
500–750ml (2–3 cups) chicken or vegetable
　stock (to make your own, see page 152)
Watercress, to serve

1. First make the salsa verde. Set aside.

2. Next, make the soup. Heat the oil in a large saucepan over a medium heat. Add the onion, garlic and leek and cook for 5–7 minutes, or until softened. Add the cauliflower florets, salt and black pepper and cook for 5 minutes, or until the cauliflower is beginning to soften.

3. Add 500ml (2 cups) of stock and bring to the boil. Reduce the heat and simmer for 5 minutes, or until the cauliflower is tender. Remove from the heat and, using a hand-held stick blender, blend until smooth. Reheat, adding more stock if you prefer a thinner soup.

4. Divide the soup between serving bowls and top with a swirl of salsa verde and watercress to serve.

Charlotte's notes

• Don't be tempted to skip the salsa verde – it really makes this soup zing. Plus, the herbs provide a source of concentrated nutrients and are important to include in your diet every day. Leftovers of this zesty dressing can be spooned over grilled chicken or fish, or used on Cauliflower pizza (page 174).

Roast squash soup *with coconut and chilli*

Cook up this vibrant vegan soup and make the most of autumnal squash. An ideal meat-free Monday lunch served with Seed and nut bread (page 136). If you're not vegan, stir a portion of roasted chicken strips through the finished soup for an extra protein boost.

Serves 4

2 tbsp extra virgin coconut oil
1 medium butternut squash (about 600g), peeled, deseeded and cut into bite-sized chunks
Pinch of sea salt
1 onion, chopped
1 leek, white part only, finely sliced
1 celery stick, finely chopped
1 garlic clove, crushed
1 red chilli, seeds removed and finely chopped, plus extra to serve

500ml (2 cups) vegetable stock (to make your own, see page 152)
250ml (1 cup) coconut milk (to make your own, see page 137)
4 tbsp sweetcorn
4 tbsp coconut cream, to serve

Serving suggestion
Seed and nut gluten-free loaf (page 136)

1. Preheat the oven to 180°C (350°F). Place the butternut squash in a roasting tin with 1 tablespoon of the coconut oil and a pinch of salt and roast for 25–30 minutes, or until soft and golden.

2. Meanwhile, melt the remaining coconut oil in a medium saucepan, add the onion, leek, celery, garlic, chilli and salt and cook over a low heat for 10–15 minutes, or until the vegetables are soft. Transfer to a blender.

3. Add the roasted butternut squash, stock and coconut milk and blend until smooth. Return to the pan, add the sweetcorn and bring back to a simmer.

4. Divide the soup between serving bowls, top with a swirl of coconut cream and sprinkle with extra chilli to serve.

Glorious green soup *with super-seedy crackers*

Broccoli takes centre stage in this vibrant green soup. Serve with fibre-rich super-seedy crackers for a fantastic crunch factor.

Serves 4

1 tbsp flavourless coconut oil

1 medium onion, finely chopped

1 garlic clove, crushed

½ tsp fennel seeds

¼ tsp sea salt

750ml (3 cups) vegetable stock

1 large head of broccoli (about 500g), chopped

½ bunch (12g) each chopped parsley, basil and chives

Coconut yoghurt and broccoli sprouts, to serve (see notes)

Cracked black pepper, for sprinkling

Super-seedy crackers

200g (1¾ cups) mixed ground flaxseed, pumpkin and sunflower seeds (see notes)

2 tbsp white chia seeds

2 tbsp sesame seeds

1 tbsp dried oregano

1 tbsp dried rosemary

2 tbsp nutritional yeast

Sea salt and cracked black pepper

1 garlic clove, crushed

Juice and zest of 1 unwaxed lemon

60ml (¼ cup) extra virgin olive oil

60ml (¼ cup) filtered water

1. Preheat the oven to 180°C (350°F). Line a large baking tray with plastic-free baking parchment.

2. To make the super-seedy crackers, place the mixed ground flaxseed, pumpkin and sunflower seeds, chia seeds, sesame seeds, oregano, rosemary, nutritional yeast, salt and black pepper in a large bowl and mix to combine.

3. Place the garlic, lemon juice and zest, oil and water in a jug and whisk to combine. Pour into the dry ingredients and mix until well combined. Pour the mixture into the prepared tray and press into a thin, even layer. Refrigerate for 15 minutes to firm up, then bake for 20 minutes. Remove from the oven and cut into rectangles. Turn the crackers over and bake for another 15–20 minutes, or until crisp.

4. Next make the soup. Heat the oil in a large saucepan over a high heat. Add the onion, garlic, fennel and salt and cook, stirring, for 3 minutes or until softened. Add the stock and bring to the boil.

5. Add the broccoli and simmer for 4–5 minutes, or until the broccoli has softened. Remove from the heat and place in a blender with the herbs. Blend until smooth and creamy.

6. Divide between serving bowls and top with a swirl of yoghurt, broccoli sprouts and a sprinkling of black pepper. Serve with the super-seedy crackers.

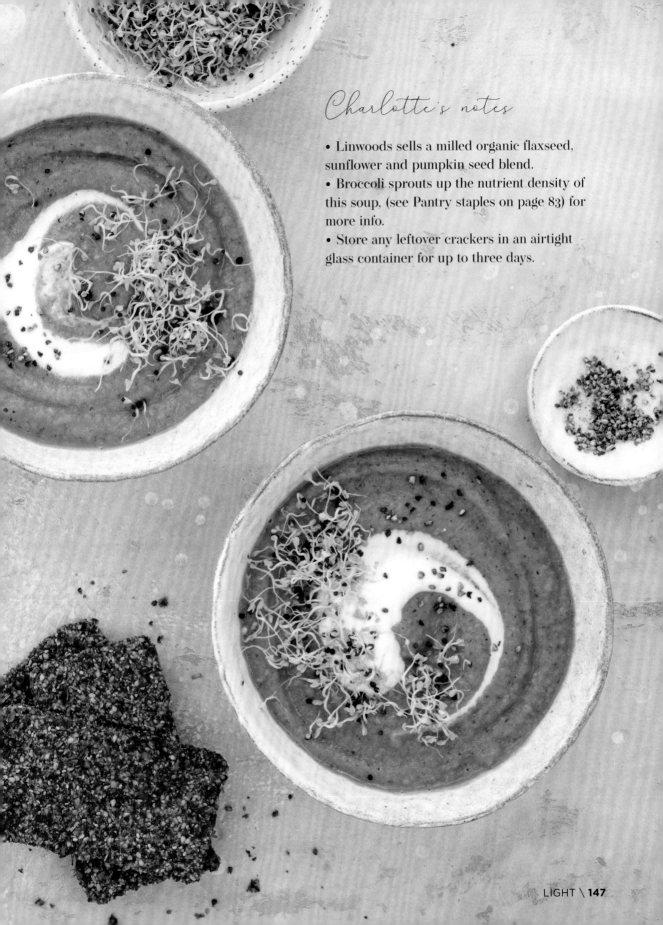

Charlotte's notes

- Linwoods sells a milled organic flaxseed, sunflower and pumpkin seed blend.
- Broccoli sprouts up the nutrient density of this soup, (see Pantry staples on page 83) for more info.
- Store any leftover crackers in an airtight glass container for up to three days.

Red miso, pak choi and crispy glazed salmon

Full of healthy fats, this crispy glazed salmon served in tangy miso broth is quick, easy and packed with flavour.

Serves 2

4 tsp sesame oil
2 x 100g salmon fillets, skin on
1 tbsp mirin (see Pantry staples on page 94)
1 tbsp tamari (see Pantry staples on page 93)
1 tsp hot chilli sauce
90g (about 3) baby pak choi, halved
   lengthways

Miso noodle broth
1 tbsp red miso paste
1 tbsp tamari
1 tbsp mirin
1 tsp finely grated ginger
750ml (3 cups) filtered water
2 courgettes, spiralised

1. First make the miso noodle broth. Place the miso paste, tamari, mirin, ginger and 125ml (½ cup) of the water in a large saucepan. Whisk until smooth. Add the remaining water and bring to a boil over a high heat. Reduce the heat and simmer for 7 minutes, adding the courgette noodles for the last minute.

2. While the broth is simmering, cook the salmon. Heat 2 teaspoons of sesame oil in a large frying pan over a high heat. Add the salmon, skin-side down, and cook for 3 minutes, or until the skin is crisp. Turn and cook for a further minute. Set aside to keep warm.

3. Place the mirin, tamari and chilli sauce in a small jug and whisk to combine. Add the remaining sesame oil to the pan and stir-fry the pak choi over a medium–high heat for 1 minute. Add the sauce and cook for a further 1–2 minutes, or until the pak choi is wilted and tender and the sauce has reduced to a syrupy glaze.

4. Divide the noodles between serving bowls and cover with the miso broth. Top with the pak choi and salmon and drizzle with the glaze to serve.

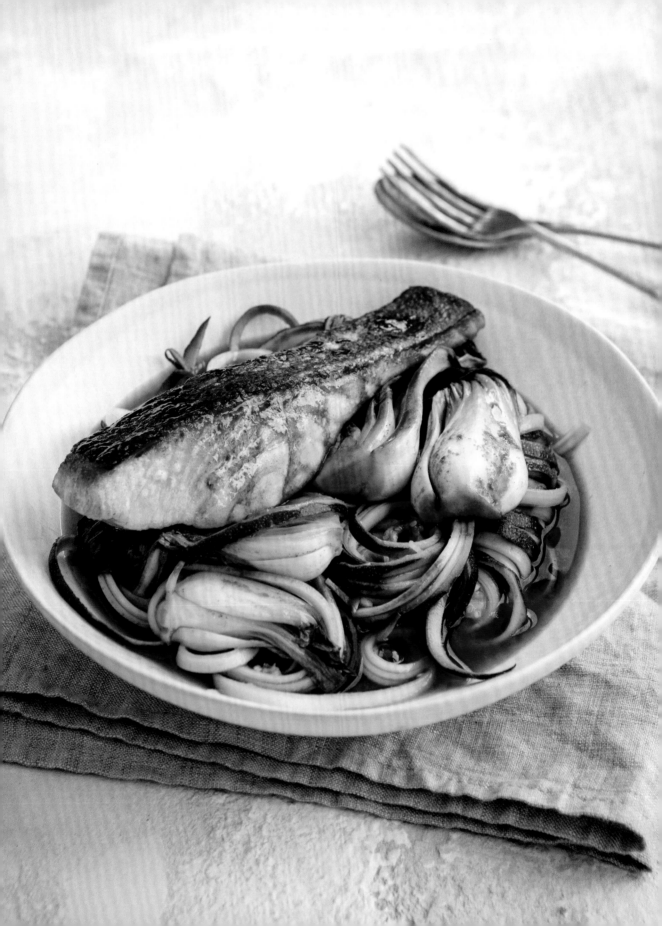

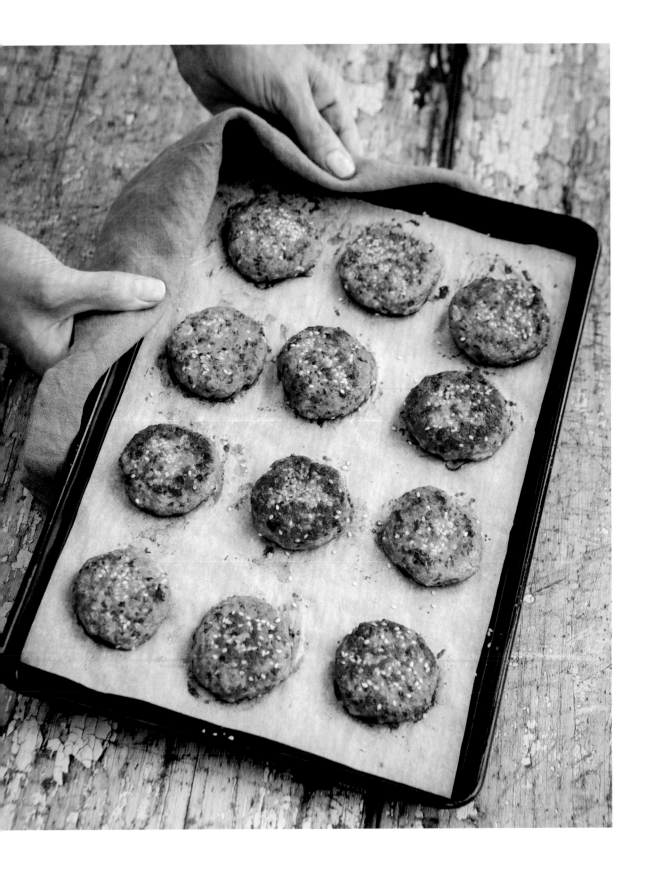

Thai salmon cakes *with chilli lime dressing*

Perfect for lunch or supper, these quick and easy salmon cakes are big on flavour.

Serves 4

1 quantity of Chilli lime dressing (page 204)
2 x 180g salmon fillets, skin and bones
    removed, roughly chopped
55g (⅓ cup) cooked quinoa
4 tbsp (35g) ground almonds
2 spring onions, thinly sliced
1 large organic free-range egg, beaten
1 garlic clove, crushed

3 tbsp chopped coriander leaves
1 tsp lemongrass paste
1 tbsp red Thai curry paste
Sesame seeds, for sprinkling
1 tbsp olive oil
Thai-style egg-fried rice (without the egg,
    page 195) and lime wedges, to serve

1. First make the chilli lime dressing. Set aside.

2. Next, make the salmon cakes. Preheat the oven to 180°C (350°F) and line a baking tray with plastic-free baking parchment. Place the salmon, quinoa, ground almonds, spring onions, egg, garlic, coriander, lemongrass paste and red Thai curry paste in a food processor and process until the mixture comes together. Using damp hands, shape the mixture into 12 patties and sprinkle with sesame seeds. Refrigerate for 5 minutes.

3. Heat the oil in a large frying pan over a medium heat. Pan-fry the patties in batches for 2–3 minutes on each side, or until golden. Transfer to the prepared tray and bake for 10 minutes, or until cooked through.

4. Serve three salmon cakes per person, on a bed of Thai-style egg-fried rice. Serve with lime wedges and a dollop of chilli lime dressing.

Charlotte's notes

• For nut-free salmon cakes, swap the almonds for ground flaxseeds.
• You can transfer leftover fish cakes to an airtight glass container and refrigerate for up to two days or freeze for up to one month. They make great lunchbox fillers.

Stocks

Stock (also known as bone broth) should be a staple in any kitchen. These simple stock recipes will add depth of flavour and goodness to a range of soups and stews.

Vegetable stock

¼ celeriac, chopped
2 large carrots, chopped
1 leek, chopped
1 large onion, chopped
3 celery sticks, chopped
½ head of fennel, chopped
1 sweet potato, chopped
¼ butternut squash, chopped
5 litres (20 cups) filtered water
2 sprigs of thyme
½ tsp salt
1 tsp black peppercorns

1. Place the vegetables in a large saucepan, cover with the water and add the thyme, salt and peppercorns. Place over a high heat, bring to the boil, then reduce the heat and simmer for 1 hour.

2. Remove from the heat and leave to stand for 2 hours. Remove the vegetables using a slotted spoon and discard them. Pass the liquid through a fine sieve into a clean glass container using a ladle. Store in the fridge for up to one week or freeze.

Chicken stock

1.2kg chicken carcass
4.5 litres (18 cups) filtered water
2 tsp sea salt
2 onions, quartered
1 leek, washed and sliced
3 celery sticks, halved
6 garlic cloves
2 tbsp chopped thyme leaves
1 tbsp black peppercorns

1. Place the chicken carcass in a large saucepan, cover with the water and add the salt. Place over a medium heat, bring to the boil, then reduce the heat and skim off the scum from the surface using a slotted spoon.

2. Add the onions, leek, celery, garlic, thyme and peppercorns. Bring back to the boil, then reduce the heat and simmer for 1 hour, carefully skimming off any more scum that rises to the surface.

3. Turn off the heat and leave to cool for 30 minutes before removing the carcass and vegetables from the pan using a small sieve or slotted spoon and discard. Strain the stock through a fine sieve into a clean glass container using a ladle. Store in the fridge for up to two days or freeze.

Fish stock

1 tbsp olive oil
1 onion, chopped
1 head of fennel, chopped
1 leek, washed and sliced
2 celery sticks, chopped
1.2kg white fish bones and trimmings,
    washed and roughly chopped
2 tbsp apple cider vinegar
1 lemon, cut into wedges
2 tbsp chopped parsley leaves
1.75 litres (7 cups) filtered water

1. Place the oil in a large saucepan over a medium heat. Stir in the onion, fennel, leek and celery and cook for 5 minutes, or until softened.

2. Add the fish bones and trimmings, apple cider vinegar, lemon wedges, parsley and water. Place over a medium heat, bring to the boil, then reduce the heat and skim off the scum from the surface using a slotted spoon.

3. Simmer for 25 minutes, carefully skimming off any more scum that rises to the surface. Turn off the heat and leave to cool for 30 minutes before removing the fish, trimmings and vegetables from the pan using a small sieve or slotted spoon and discard. Strain the stock through a fine sieve into a clean glass container using a ladle. Store in the fridge for up to two days or freeze.

Boosted stock
(fresh ginger and turmeric)

This immunity boosting stock can be drunk as a daily tonic to support gut health and to keep those winter colds at bay.

250ml (1 cup) chicken stock
Juice of 1 lemon
Pinch of cayenne
1 tsp grated ginger
1 tsp grated turmeric
Slice of lemon

Place the chicken stock, lemon juice, cayenne, ginger and turmeric in a small saucepan over a high heat. Bring to the boil, then turn off the heat and steep for 5 minutes. Strain into a cup and add a slice of lemon to serve.

Rainbow jar salad
with green goddess dressing

This jar salad is always a hit with my clients – eating the rainbow has never been simpler. Easy to prep ahead and portable, this jar salad is sure to become a working-lunch staple.

Serve 1

Handful of raw walnuts, or other nuts or seeds of your choice
½ candied beetroot, chopped
½ small courgette, spiralised or julienned (cut into matchsticks)
Rocket or salad leaves of your choice

Handful of cherry tomatoes, halved
1 portion of protein of your choice (I used Tandoori salmon, page 163)
1 small carrot, grated or julienned
4 tbsp Green goddess dressing (page 205)

1. Layer all the salad ingredients in a large glass jar.

2. Make the green goddess dressing. Drizzle over the salad just before serving.

Charlotte's notes

• The beauty of this salad is that you can use whatever salad vegetables you prefer – just go for as many different colours as possible. Always include a portion of protein, such as roasted chicken strips, tandoori salmon, mackerel, egg or cooked chickpeas, and a healthy fat such as nuts, seeds or avocado.
• If you have time, you can try out different techniques to add interest to your salad; I like to use a serrated knife, or grate, julienne or cube my veggies. When food looks pretty it's so much more tempting!
• Leftover green goddess dressing will keep in an airtight container in the fridge for up to two days. It tastes amazing drizzled on baked veggies.

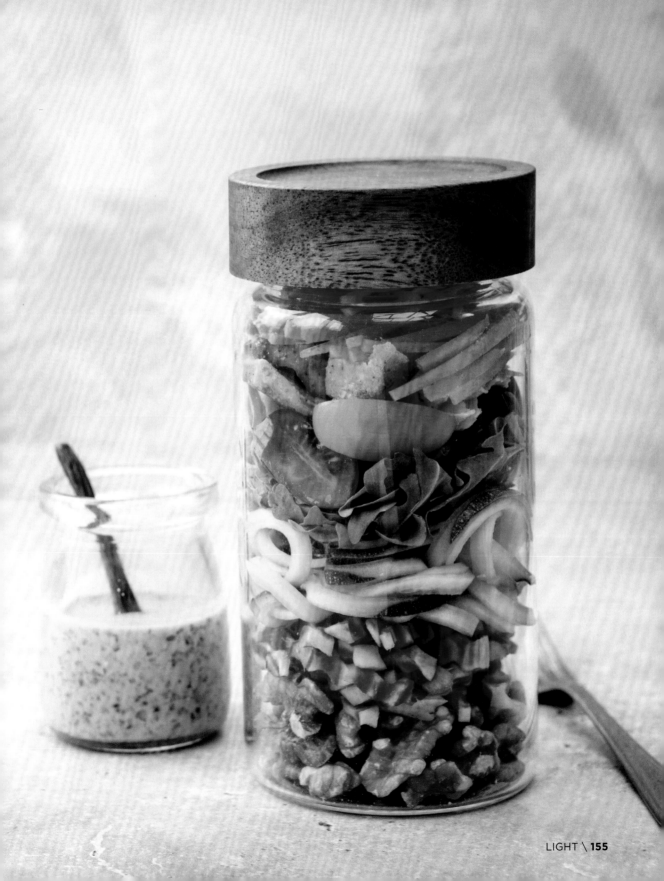

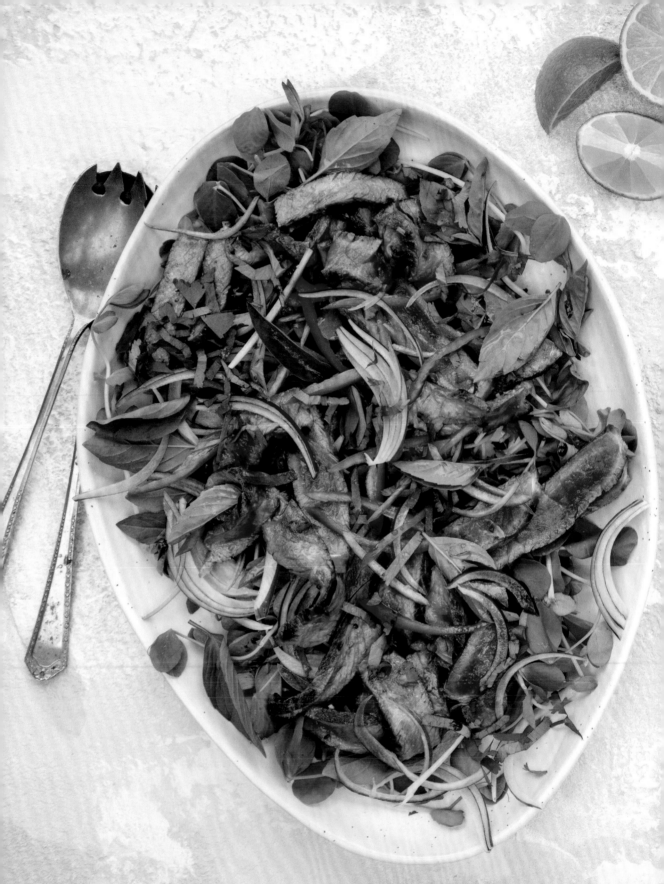

Thai beef salad

This beef is infused with delicious Thai flavours. This will become your go-to salad when you're craving iron.

Serves 2

2 x 180g grass-fed fillet steaks
Sesame oil, for brushing
1 small red onion, finely sliced
1 long red chilli, deseeded and sliced into matchsticks
40g (1 cup, tightly packed) pea shoots
½ bunch (12g) Thai basil leaves
½ bunch (12g) coriander leaves
Lime wedges, to serve

For the marinade

1 tsp sea salt
1 garlic clove, crushed
1 tbsp grated ginger
1½ tsp tamari or coconut aminos (see notes)
½ tsp sesame oil
2 tbsp rice vinegar
2 tsp raw honey

1. First make the marinade. Place all the ingredients in a large bowl and whisk to combine. Add the steaks, toss to coat and place in the fridge for 1 hour, or overnight, to marinate.

2. Heat a large frying pan over a high heat. Remove the steaks from the marinade, pat dry and brush with sesame oil. Cook the steaks for 2–3 minutes each side for medium-rare, or until cooked to your liking. Set aside for 5 minutes to rest, then thinly slice.

3. To make the salad, place the onion, chilli, pea shoots, Thai basil and coriander in a medium bowl and toss lightly.

4. Toss the beef through the salad and serve with lime wedges.

Charlotte's notes

• Thai basil has an anise-like, slightly spicy flavour.
• Tamari is gluten-free soy sauce. If you are avoiding soy, use coconut aminos (see Pantry staples on page 86).

Roasted butternut, tomato and Puy lentil salad

A rustic and warming super-healthy salad with lemon and mustard dressing and lots of folate-rich baby leaf spinach.

Serves 2

½ small butternut squash (about 250g), peeled, deseeded and sliced
Olive oil, for brushing
Sea salt and cracked black pepper
1 small red onion, thinly sliced
1 tbsp white wine vinegar
Pinch sea salt
1 quantity of Lemon mustard dressing (page 205)

125g (½ cup) cooked Puy lentils
50g (⅓ cup) radishes, thinly sliced
90g (2 cups, tightly packed) baby leaf spinach
½ bunch (12g) dill, roughly chopped
2 medium tomatoes, sliced

1. Preheat the oven to 200°C (400°F). Line a baking tray with plastic-free baking parchment.

2. Place the butternut squash on the baking tray and brush with the oil. Season with salt and black pepper. Roast for 30–35 minutes, or until tender and golden, turning once and brushing with oil halfway through cooking.

3. Place the onion in a small bowl, toss with the white wine vinegar and salt and set aside for 5–10 minutes to marinate.

4. Meanwhile, make the lemon mustard dressing. Set aside.

5. To assemble the salad, combine the roasted butternut squash, lentils, radishes, spinach, onions and most of the dill in a medium bowl.

6. Divide the salad between serving plates and top with the tomatoes. Drizzle with the dressing and scatter with the remaining dill to serve.

Charlotte's notes

Leftover butternut squash can be used in the Roast squash soup with coconut and chilli (page 145). Otherwise, slice and freeze it for use another time.

Chicken Caesar *with smoky chickpeas and soft-boiled eggs*

This chicken Caesar salad is next level nutritious and delicious, featuring chargrilled chicken, smoky chickpeas, soft-boiled eggs and a creamy mustard dressing.

Serves 2

1 tsp finely grated unwaxed lemon zest

1 tbsp tarragon leaves, finely chopped, plus extra to serve

2 tbsp olive oil

Sea salt and cracked black pepper

1 x 180g organic free-range chicken breast fillet

2 large organic free-range eggs

1 quantity of Caesar dressing (page 205)

2 tbsp pumpkin seeds

2 baby cos (romaine) lettuces, trimmed

2 carrots, grated

For the smoky chickpeas

1 x 350g jar chickpeas, drained and rinsed

1 tbsp olive oil

¼ tsp sea salt

½ tsp Italian seasoning

¼ tsp garlic powder

¼ tsp smoked paprika

1. First, make the marinade for the chicken. Place the lemon zest, tarragon, oil, salt, black pepper and chicken in a medium bowl and toss to coat. Set aside.

2. Place the eggs in a small saucepan of boiling water for 5–6 minutes, or until soft boiled. Refresh in iced water, peel, halve and set aside.

3. Preheat a chargrill pan over a medium heat. Cook the chicken for 6–8 minutes each side, or until cooked through. Slice and set aside.

4. Meanwhile, make the Caesar dressing. Set aside.

5. To make the smoky chickpeas, place the chickpeas in a medium pan with the oil, salt, Italian seasoning, garlic powder and smoked paprika and cook over a medium–high heat for 3–4 minutes, or until fully coated and warmed through. Remove the chickpeas from the pan and set aside to cool.

6. Place the pumpkin seeds in the same pan and heat on a medium–high heat for 2–3 minutes, or until slightly golden. Set aside.

7. Divide the lettuces, carrots, eggs, chicken, chickpeas and pumpkin seeds between serving plates. Drizzle with the dressing and sprinkle with extra tarragon and black pepper to serve.

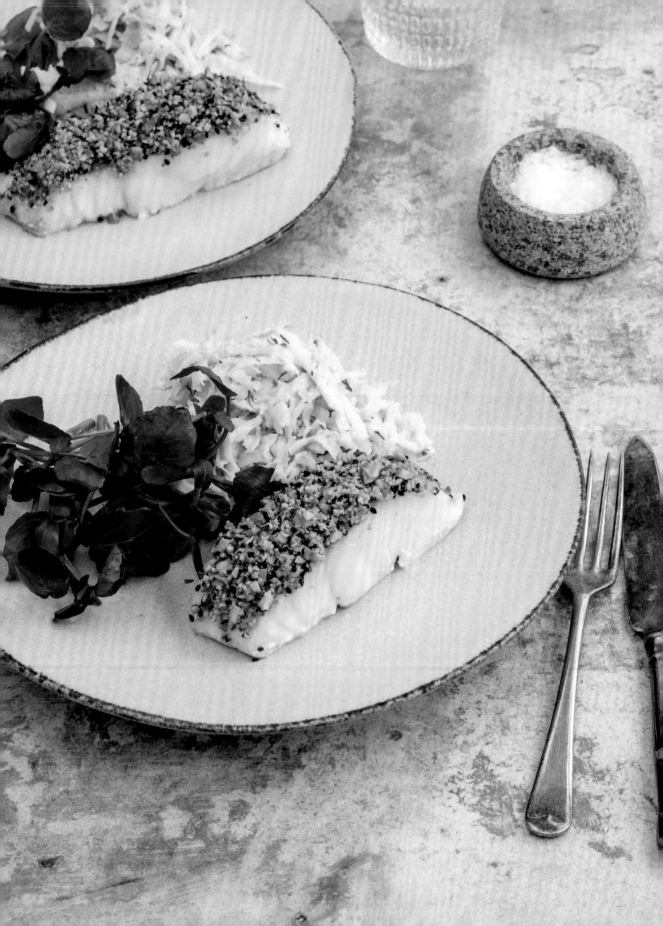

Green dukkah-crusted cod *with celeriac slaw*

Dukkah pairs perfectly with this mild fish. Delicate, flaky cod is a great fish to add into your diet.

Serves 2

2 tbsp extra virgin olive oil

2 x 100g (3½ oz) skinless wild cod fillets, about 2.5cm (1 inch) thick

60g (¼ cup) coconut yoghurt

¾ tsp Dijon mustard

1 tsp dried dill

Juice of ½ lemon

Sea salt and cracked black pepper

½ small celeriac (about 150g), peeled and coarsely grated

60g (2 cups) watercress and lemon wedges, to serve

For the green dukkah

150g (1 cup) almonds

150g (1 cup) pistachios

3 tbsp black sesame seeds

2 tbsp green fennel seeds

Pinch of sea salt

1. Preheat the oven to 180°C (350°F). Line two baking trays with plastic-free baking parchment.

2. First, make the green dukkah. Arrange the almonds and pistachios in an even layer on one of the prepared trays. Roast for 8 minutes, shaking the tray once halfway through cooking. Leave to cool completely. Meanwhile, dry-fry the seeds in a pan over a heat high for 3 minutes, tossing constantly. Leave to cool completely. Place the cooled nuts and seeds with the salt in a pestle and mortar and grind until finely chopped (alternatively, use a food processor).

3. Put the oil and 2 tablespoons of the dukkah in a small bowl and mix to combine. Place the fish on the baking tray and spoon half the dukkah and oil mixture onto each fillet, pressing firmly into the flesh. Bake for 12 minutes, or until the fish flakes easily when tested with a fork.

4. While the fish is cooking, place the yoghurt, mustard, dill and lemon juice in a medium bowl and whisk to combine. Season with salt and black pepper. Toss the celeriac in the dressing.

5. Divide the watercress between serving plates, top with the celeriac slaw and cod and serve with lemon wedges.

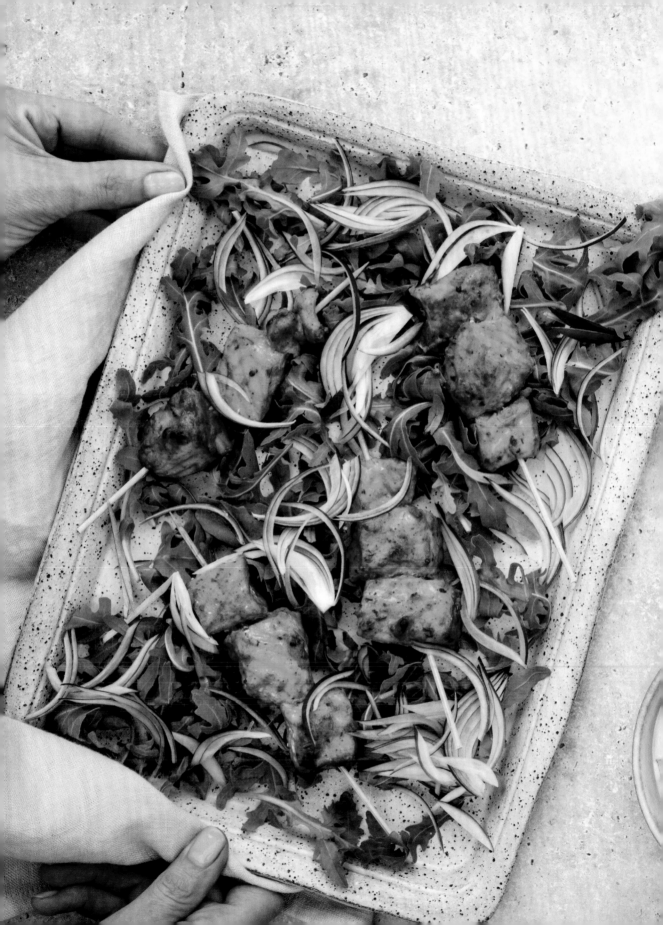

Tandoori salmon skewers *with raita and onion salad*

Tandoori combines all the wonderful flavours of India in a spicy, fruity, smoky and deliciously intense blend. If you're new to eating oily fish or are not usually a fan, this is a great recipe to start with, as the tandoori flavour dominates.

Serves 2

80g (⅓ cup) coconut yoghurt
1½ tsp tandoori masala curry blend
2 x 110g wild Alaskan or sockeye boneless
  salmon fillets, skins removed and cut
  into chunks
Rocket, lime wedges and 1 small red onion,
  finely sliced, to serve

For the raita
¼ small cucumber, seeds removed and sliced
2 tbsp coconut yoghurt
Juice of ½ lime
2 sprigs of mint, leaves removed and
  finely chopped
Pinch of salt

1. Preheat the grill to medium–high. Put the coconut yoghurt and tandoori masala curry blend in a small bowl and whisk until smooth. Add the salmon chunks, coating them well and set aside to marinate.

2. Next, make the raita. Place the cucumber in a small bowl with the coconut yoghurt, lime juice, mint and salt and mix to combine. Set aside.

3. Thread the salmon onto 4 skewers and grill for 2–3 minutes on each side. Divide the raita between serving plates and top each with 2 skewers, a handful of rocket and a lime wedge. Sprinkle with the onion to serve.

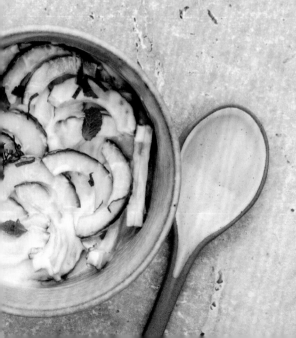

Charlotte's notes

For even bolder flavour, marinate the salmon overnight. If you are using wooden skewers, soak them in water for at least 20 minutes before use so that they don't burn.

Pan-fried Asian-style mackerel
with aubergine and cavolo nero

This no-fuss meal is packed with Asian flavours of sweet, salty teriyaki sauce.

Serves 2

2 small aubergines, cut into 1.5cm-thick rounds
2 x 180g Atlantic mackerel fillets
1 tbsp sesame oil
1 spring onion, finely sliced
1 tsp grated ginger
1 garlic clove, crushed
150g (5 cups) cavolo nero, stalks removed and leaves roughly chopped

Sesame seeds and 1 spring onion, finely sliced, to serve

For the teriyaki marinade
60ml (¼ cup) tamari
2 tsp sesame oil
1 tsp honey
1 tsp grated ginger
1 tsp Dijon mustard

1. Preheat the grill to high. Grease a ceramic or glass ovenproof dish.

2. First make the teriyaki marinade. Place all the ingredients in a small bowl and whisk to combine. Spread the aubergine slices and mackerel fillets in a shallow dish and pour over the marinade, leaving to soak for 2 minutes.

3. Arrange the aubergine slices on the prepared dish and grill for 5–6 minutes on each side, or until tender and golden brown. Baste with the marinade on both sides when turning.

4. Heat 1½ teaspoons of the sesame oil in a large frying pan over a medium heat and stir-fry the spring onion, ginger and garlic for 2–3 minutes, or until fragrant. Add the cavolo nero and stir-fry for a further 2 minutes.

5. Next, cook the fish. Heat the remaining sesame oil in a small frying pan over a medium–high heat and sear the mackerel, skin-side down, for 1–2 minutes. Turn the fish over, add the remaining marinade to the pan and cook for a further 1–2 minutes, or until the fish is cooked through.

6. Divide the cavolo nero between serving plates, top with the aubergine slices and mackerel and drizzle over any leftover marinade from the pan. Sprinkle with the sesame seeds and spring onion to serve.

Mediterranean roast veggie ragù

Serve this delicious one-pan vegan ragù for an easy,
fuss-free midweek dinner.

Serves 4

2½ tsp Italian seasoning
½ tsp sea salt
¼ tsp cracked black pepper
2 tbsp olive oil
3 large garlic cloves, crushed
2 medium courgettes, chopped into bite-sized
   chunks
1 red pepper, chopped into bite-sized chunks
14 mixed cherry tomatoes, halved
6 baby new potatoes, halved
1 large red onion, chopped into chunks

1 x 325g jar butter beans, drained and rinsed
1 x 680g jar passata rustica
2 tbsp tomato purée
100g kalamata olives, stones removed
   and halved
1 bunch (25g) basil leaves, roughly chopped
2 tbsp pine nuts and 4 tsp nutritional yeast,
   to serve

1. Preheat the oven to 180°C (350°F).

2. Place the Italian seasoning, salt, black pepper, oil and garlic in a large
bowl and whisk to combine. Add the courgettes, red pepper, cherry
tomatoes, potatoes, onion and butter beans and toss to coat well.

3. Spread the vegetables evenly in a roasting tin and place in the oven for
30–35 minutes, or until the vegetables are golden and tender, tossing once
halfway through. Add the passata and tomato purée, mix well to combine
and return to the oven for 5 minutes.

4. Remove from the oven and stir through the olives and basil. Divide the
ragù between serving bowls and sprinkle with the pine nuts and 1 teaspoon
of nutritional yeast per person to serve.

Charlotte's notes

Leftover ragù will keep in an airtight glass container in the fridge for
up to three days or in the freezer for up to one month.

Yellow coconut curry *with tiger prawns*

Serve up this healthy prawn curry with vibrant turmeric, ginger and coconut flavours for an easy, delicious midweek meal.

Serves 2

1 lemongrass stalk, trimmed and very finely chopped
2 tsp brown mustard seeds (see Pantry staples on page 83)
½ tsp ground cardamom
1 tsp ground turmeric
1 onion, finely sliced
1 bunch (25g) coriander stalks, finely chopped
2 tsp grated ginger
2 garlic cloves, crushed
½ tsp sea salt
2–3 tbsp filtered water

1 tbsp extra virgin coconut oil
½ small butternut squash (about 300g), peeled, deseeded and cut into 1cm dice
6 baby corns, thinly sliced into rounds
400ml (1¾ cups) coconut milk (to make your own, see page 137)
½ small pineapple (about 200g), peeled, cored and cut into chunks

10–12 pre-cooked extra-large tiger prawns (about 150g)
1 bunch (25g) coriander leaves, roughly chopped, to serve

Serving suggestion
Thai-style egg-fried rice (without the egg, page 195)

1. First make a curry paste. Place the lemongrass, mustard seeds, cardamom and turmeric in a wok over a medium–high heat and dry-fry for 1–2 minutes, or until fragrant. Transfer to a small food processor with the onion, coriander stalks, ginger, garlic, salt and 2 tablespoons of the water. Process to a smooth consistency, adding another tablespoon of water to thin if needed.

2. Next, make the curry. Heat the oil in the same wok over a medium–high heat. Add the paste and cook for 3–4 minutes, or until fragrant. Add the butternut squash and corn and stir to coat in the paste and when nicely coloured add the coconut milk and pineapple, cover and bring to a boil. Reduce the heat and simmer for 15 minutes, or until the squash is just tender.

3. Stir in the prawns and cook for 3–4 minutes, or until warmed through. Divide between serving bowls and sprinkle with the chopped coriander to serve.

Charlotte's notes

Leftover curry will keep in an airtight glass container in the fridge for up to two days.

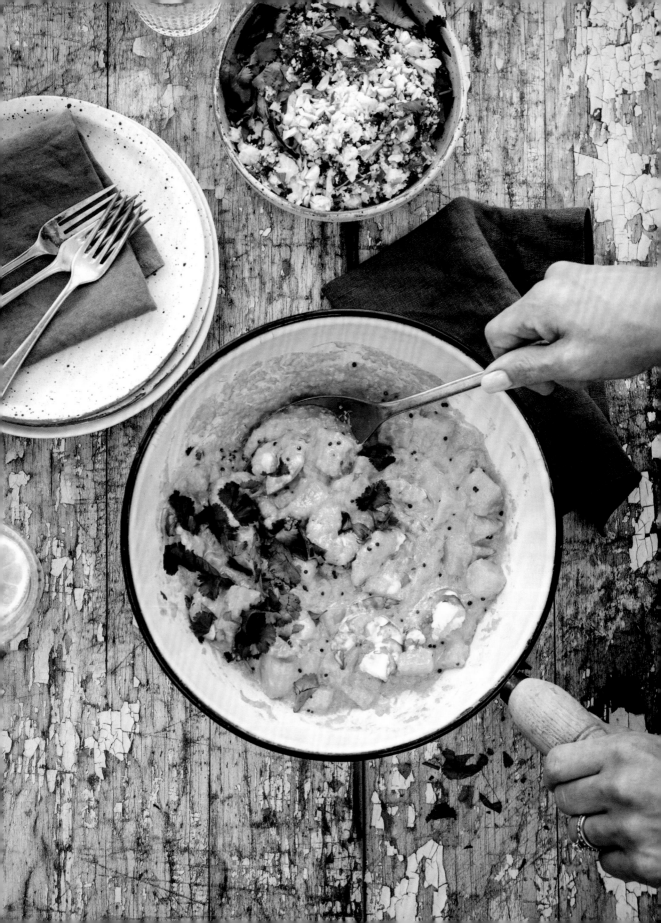

Slow-cooked beef and black bean chilli

This veg-packed chilli is an easy weekday meal, as you can set it and forget it. The slow-cooker method results in flavour-infused beef that melts in the mouth. Don't leave the liver out because it provides a nutrient boost and will be well hidden in this recipe.

Serves 6

2 tbsp olive oil
2 medium onions, finely chopped
2 celery sticks, finely chopped
2 medium carrots, coarsely grated
1 medium courgette, coarsely grated
1 red pepper, cut into bite-sized chunks
2 garlic cloves, crushed
1 tsp ground cumin
1 tsp paprika

½ tsp hot chilli powder
½ tsp sea salt
¼ tsp cracked black pepper
500g grass-fed beef steak mince
100g organic free-range chicken livers, puréed
1 x 680g jar passata rustica
2 tbsp tomato purée
1 tbsp red miso paste (optional, see Pantry staples on page 91)
1 tbsp sherry vinegar (see Pantry staples on page 94)

60ml (¼ cup) chicken or vegetable stock (to make your own, see page 152)
14 cherry tomatoes, halved
1 x 350g jar black beans, drained and rinsed

To serve
Coconut yoghurt
1 avocado, chopped into bite-sized chunks
Coriander leaves, roughly chopped
Lime wedges

1. Gently heat the oil in a large, deep frying pan over a medium heat. Add the onions, celery, carrots, courgette, red pepper, garlic, cumin, paprika, chilli powder, salt and black pepper and cook for 5 minutes, or until the vegetables are just beginning to soften. Increase the heat to high, add the mince and cook for 3–4 minutes, or until browned, breaking up any lumps with a wooden spoon.

2. Transfer to a slow cooker and add the chicken livers, passata, tomato purée, miso paste (if using), sherry vinegar and chicken or vegetable stock and stir well to combine.

3. Cover and cook on low for 7–8 hours or high for 4 hours. Add the cherry tomatoes and black beans and cook on high, uncovered, for 20 minutes, or until thickened.

4. Divide the chilli between serving bowls and top with yoghurt and avocado. Sprinkle with coriander and serve with lime wedges.

Easy weeknight curry

Forget ordering takeaway and make this tasty vegan curry instead. It's quick, healthy and full of flavour. Batch cook and freeze leftovers for another day.

Serves 4

1 onion, diced
2 garlic cloves, crushed
Thumb-sized piece of ginger, finely grated
1 bunch (25g) coriander stalks, finely chopped
2 tsp garam masala
2 tsp ground coriander
1 tsp ground turmeric
1 tsp ground cumin
1 tsp sea salt
½ tsp hot chilli powder
2–3 tbsp filtered water
1 tbsp coconut oil

1 small head of cauliflower (about 300g), chopped into florets
1 medium sweet potato (about 225g), peeled and cut into bite-sized chunks
250g (1 cup) passata rustica
250ml (1 cup) full-fat coconut milk
350g jar chickpeas, drained and rinsed
135g (3 cups, tightly packed) spinach
70g (½ cup) whole cashews
1 bunch (25g) coriander leaves, roughly chopped, to serve

1. First make a curry paste. Place the onion, garlic, ginger, coriander stalks, garam masala, coriander, turmeric, cumin, salt, chilli powder and 2 tablespoons of the water in a small food processor and process to a paste, adding another tablespoon of water to thin if needed.

2. Next, make the curry. Heat the oil in a large saucepan over a medium–high heat, add the curry paste and cook, stirring occasionally, for 2–3 minutes, or until fragrant.

3. Add the cauliflower and sweet potato and stir to coat in the paste. When nicely coloured add the passata, coconut milk and chickpeas and stir to combine. Cover, bring to a boil, then reduce the heat to low and cook, stirring occasionally, for 15–20 minutes, or until the sauce is slightly thickened and the vegetables have softened. Top the curry with the spinach and leave to wilt for 2–3 minutes before stirring through.

4. Meanwhile, dry-fry the cashews over a high heat for 3–4 minutes, or until golden brown, tossing frequently. Leave to cool, then roughly chop.

5. Spoon the curry into serving bowls and sprinkle with the toasted cashews and coriander leaves to serve.

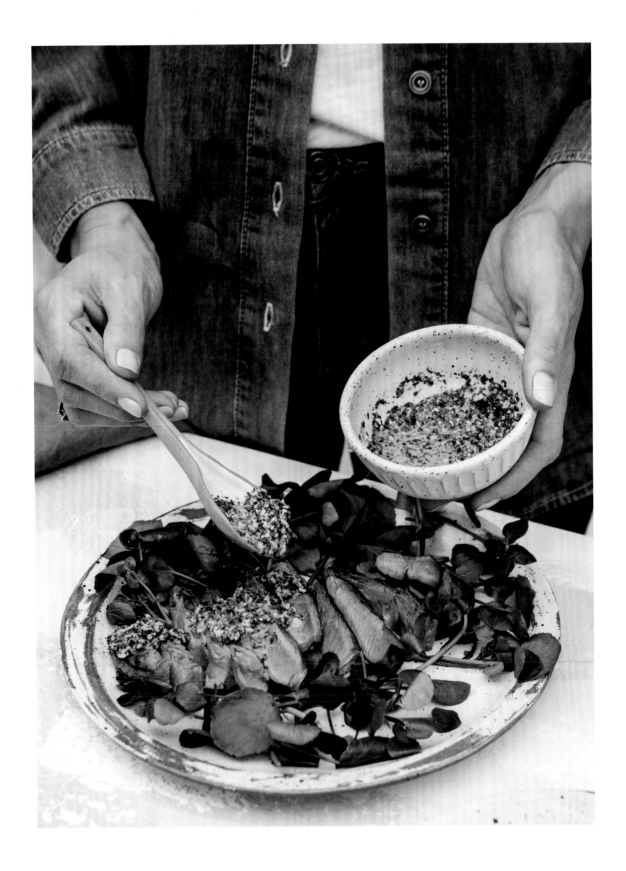

Steak with chimichurri sauce

Indulge in rib-eye steak topped with vibrant chimichurri for a simple Friday-night supper. Why not boost your veg intake by making Veggie mash (page 194) to go alongside?

Serves 2

2 x 125g organic grass-fed rib-eye or sirloin steaks
Flavourless coconut oil
Sea salt and cracked black pepper
60g (2 cups, tightly packed) watercress, to serve

For the chimichurri sauce
3 tbsp pumpkin seeds
60ml (¼ cup) filtered water
28g (1 cup) coriander or parsley
2 tbsp sherry vinegar (see Pantry staples on page 94)
2 tbsp extra virgin olive oil
1 garlic clove, crushed
½ tsp dried oregano
½ tsp salt

1. Rub the steaks with oil, season with salt and black pepper and set aside.

2. Next make the chimichurri sauce. Place the pumpkin seeds in a small food processor and process until the seeds are finely ground. Add the water, coriander, sherry vinegar, oil, garlic, oregano and salt and pulse to a chunky paste consistency.

3. To cook the steaks, heat a griddle pan over a medium–high heat and cook for 2–3 minutes on each side, or until done to your liking. Leave to rest for a few minutes.

4. Slice the steaks, divide between serving plates and spoon over the chimichurri. Serve with the watercress.

Charlotte's notes

• If you don't have sherry vinegar, use red wine vinegar instead.
• Leftover chimichurri will keep in an airtight glass container in the fridge for up to two days.

Lemon-and-herb-crusted roast chicken

This one-tray, easy roast chicken is bursting with flavour thanks to fresh herbs, lemon and garlic. It makes a tasty Sunday lunch to enjoy with friends.

Serves 6

1 whole organic free-range chicken (about 1.4kg)*
25g (½ cup) herbs (sage, rosemary and thyme), roughly chopped, plus an extra sprig of each for the chicken cavity
Zest, finely grated, and juice of 1 lemon (reserve the lemon halves for the chicken cavity)
1 red onion, quartered
8 baby carrots, trimmed

1 cauliflower, cut into florets
1 medium sweet potato, chopped into chunks
Olive oil, for drizzling
Sea salt and cracked black pepper
125ml (½ cup) flavourless coconut oil or organic grass-fed butter, softened
3 garlic cloves, crushed
Steamed greens, to serve

1. Preheat oven to 190°C (375°F).

2. Set the chicken in the centre of a large roasting tin and place the herb sprigs and lemon halves inside the chicken cavity. Add the onion, carrots, cauliflower and sweet potato to the pan, drizzle with olive oil and season with salt and black pepper.

3. Place the softened coconut oil, chopped herbs, lemon zest and juice, garlic, and 1 teaspoon of salt and black pepper each in a small bowl and mix to combine. Using your hands, loosen the skin from the flesh of the chicken and evenly spread half the lemon and herb mixture under the skin. Spread the remaining mixture over the top of the chicken, covering all the skin.

4. Roast for 1 hour 20 minutes, or until the chicken is golden brown and the juices run clear when tested with a skewer. If the chicken gets too brown, loosely tent with parchment paper for the remainder of the cooking time. Remove from the oven, loosely tent with parchment and leave to rest for 10 minutes before carving. Serve with the vegetables and greens.

*Allow 20 minutes per 500g + 20 minutes' cooking time (until the juices run clear).

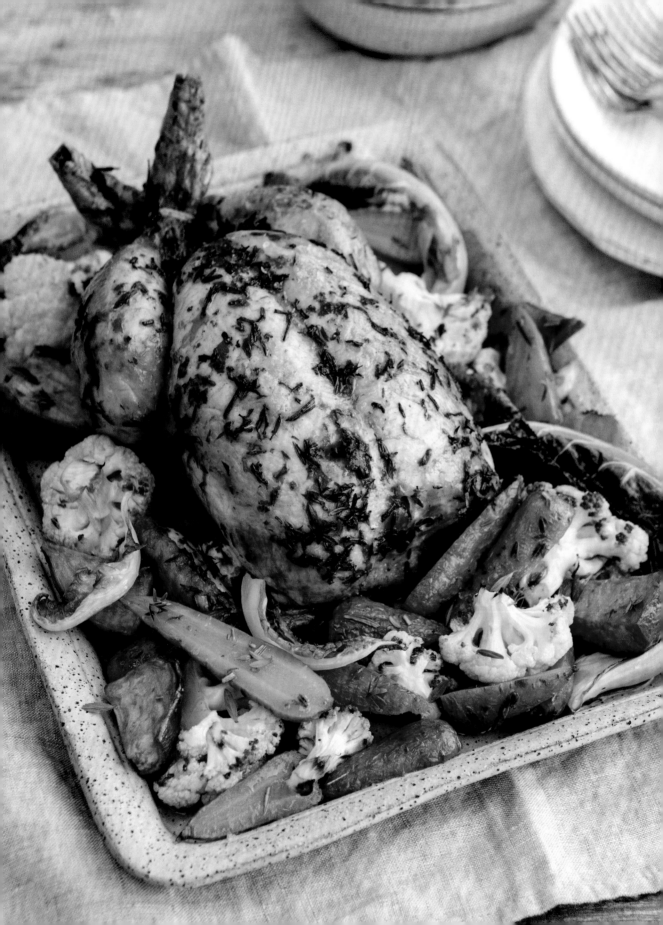

Green goddess cauliflower pizza

Up your pizza game with this cauliflower base variation. It is truly delicious and a great way to pack in extra vegetables.

Serves 2

For the cauliflower pizza bases

1 large cauliflower (about 600g), cut into florets (stems discarded)
90g (³/4 cup) ground almonds
30g (¹/4 cup) ground flaxseeds
3 large organic free-range eggs, beaten

2 tbsp nutritional yeast flakes (see Pantry staples on page 91), plus extra for sprinkling
1 tbsp Italian herbs mix
Sea salt and cracked black pepper

Toppings

1 quantity of Salsa verde (page 209)
1 courgette, cut into ribbons

55g (¹/2 cup) chargrilled artichoke chunks (see Pantry stapes on page 82)
60g (¹/2 cup) plant-based mozzarella, torn (or use buffalo mozzarella if tolerated)
Olive oil, for drizzling
2 handfuls of watercress, to serve

1. Preheat the oven to 180°C (350°F). Lightly grease and line two 30cm round pizza trays with plastic-free baking parchment.

2. First make the pizza bases. Place the cauliflower in a food processor and process until the mixture resembles fine breadcrumbs. Transfer to a clean tea towel and squeeze out as much moisture as possible. Add to a large bowl with the ground almonds, ground flaxseeds, eggs, nutritional yeast, Italian herbs mix, salt and black pepper and mix to form a soft dough.

3. Divide the mixture in half, gently press into 25cm circles on the prepared trays and bake for 20–25 minutes, or until golden and crispy.

4. Now make the salsa verde. Set aside.

5. Remove the pizza bases from the oven, leave to cool slightly, then loosen from the parchment with a palette knife. Spread with a thin layer of salsa verde, reserving some to drizzle on the pizzas after baking, and add the courgette, artichokes and mozzarella. Drizzle with olive oil and return the pizzas to the oven for another 8–10 minutes.

6. Allow to cool slightly before drizzling each pizza with the reserved salsa verde. Top with watercress and sprinkle with nutritional yeast.

Cauliflower pizza variations
• Try homemade Failproof tomato sauce (page 208) instead of salsa verde.
• For a super-green pizza base, swap the cauliflower for broccoli.

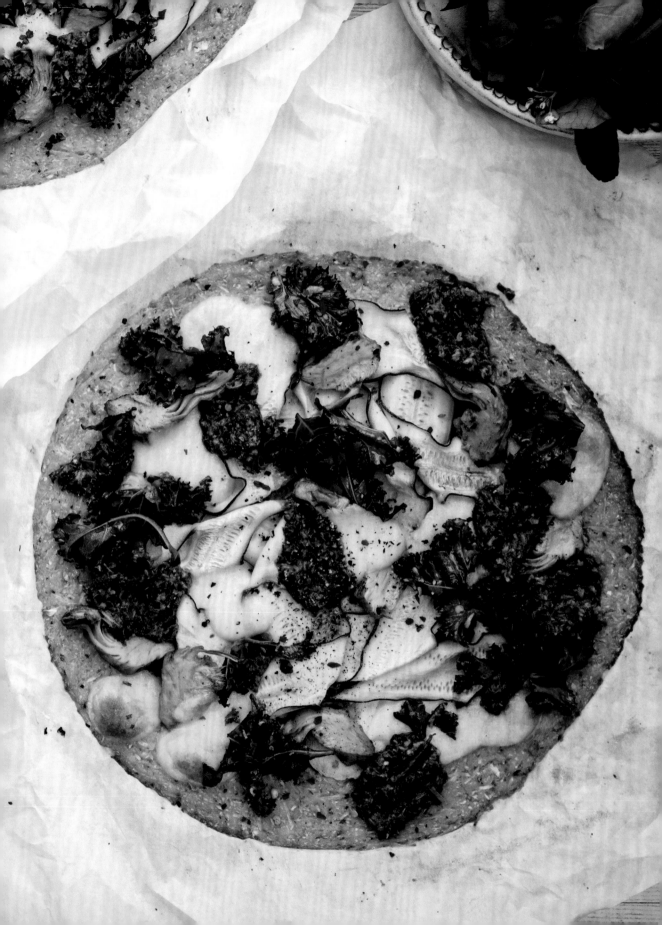

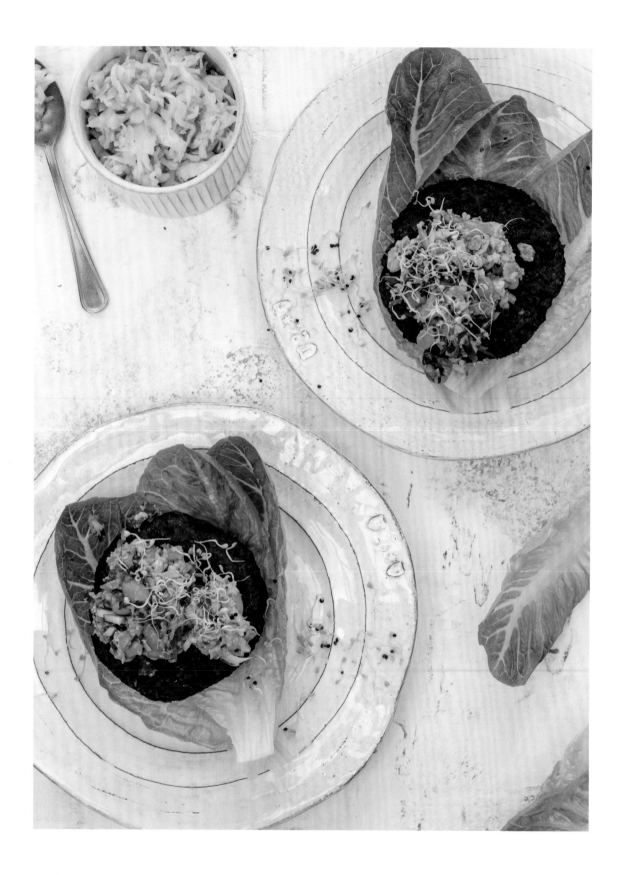

Beetroot burgers *with avocado and edamame smash*

These hearty beet (not beef!) burgers are loaded with flavour and will satisfy even the most dedicated of meat eaters!

Serves 2

1 tsp olive oil, plus extra for brushing
1 small onion, grated
1 garlic clove, crushed
100g (1 medium) beetroot, peeled and grated
45g (⅓ cup) ground walnuts
3 tbsp ground flaxseeds
1 large organic free-range egg

1 tbsp chopped flat-leaf parsley
½ tsp ground cumin
½ tsp ground coriander
Sea salt and cracked black pepper

1 quantity of Avocado and edamame smash (page 202)

To serve
4 large pieces of romaine lettuce
Broccoli sprouts (see Pantry staples on page 83)
Sauerkraut (to make your own, see page 191)

1. Preheat the oven to 180°C (350°F). Line a baking tray with plastic-free baking parchment.

2. First make the burgers. Heat the oil in a small frying pan over a medium heat. Add the onion and garlic and cook for 4–5 minutes, or until softened. Transfer to a food processor and add the beetroot, ground walnuts, ground flaxseeds, egg, parsley, cumin, coriander, salt and black pepper and pulse until just combined. Shape into 2 large burger patties and refrigerate for at least 15 minutes to firm up.

3. Next, make the avocado and edamame smash. Set aside.

4. Remove the burgers from the fridge and brush with oil. Cook in the oven for 25–30 minutes, or until golden brown, turning once and brushing with more oil halfway through cooking.

5. To assemble the burgers, lay down a piece of romaine lettuce on each serving plate. Top with a dollop of avocado and edamame smash, a handful of broccoli sprouts, a burger and sauerkraut, finishing with another piece of romaine to make a lettuce bun.

Beef burgers *with avocado and edamame smash*

These beef burgers offer another great way to add nutrient-rich liver into your diet. Serve these succulent burgers with avocado and edamame smash for an easy midweek meal.

Serves 2

220g organic grass-fed beef mince
30g organic chicken liver, finely grated (see notes)
1 small onion, finely chopped
1 garlic clove, minced
1 tsp ground cumin
1 tsp ground coriander
Sea salt and cracked black pepper
2 tsp olive oil

1 quantity of Avocado and edamame smash (page 202)

To serve
4 large pieces of romaine lettuce
Broccoli sprouts (see Pantry staples on page 83)
Sauerkraut (to make your own, see page 191)

1. First make the meat patties. Place the mince, liver, onion, garlic, cumin, coriander, salt and black pepper in a large bowl and mix until well combined. Divide the mixture equally and shape into 2 large patties.

2. Heat the oil in a large non-stick frying pan over a medium heat. Add the patties and cook for 4–5 minutes each side, or until browned and cooked through.

3. While the burgers are cooking, make the avocado and edamame smash. Set aside.

4. To assemble the burgers, lay down a piece of romaine lettuce on each serving plate. Top with a dollop of avocado and edamame smash, a handful of broccoli sprouts, a burger and sauerkraut, finishing with another piece of romaine to make a lettuce bun.

Charlotte's notes

• Liver is easier to grate if you freeze it first.
• Why not double the quantities and once you have made the burger patties, shape and cook 6 smaller patties to enjoy cold for lunch another day? Cook once, eat twice!

Slow-cooked pulled pork *with cauliflower cream*

I've jazzed up pulled pork with a sweet and fragrant spice blend that smells insane when cooking! Share this deeply satisfying weekend showstopper with some lucky friends.

Serves 6–8

1 tbsp ground black pepper
1 tbsp ground allspice
1 tbsp ground cinnamon
1 tsp ground nutmeg
1 tsp ground coriander
1 tsp ground cumin
1 tsp ground cloves
1–1.5kg free-range pork shoulder (preferably bone in)

2 tsp olive oil, for greasing
2 bay leaves
80ml (1/3 cup) chicken stock
80ml (1/3 cup) apple cider vinegar
190g (3/4 cup) passata rustica
2 garlic cloves, crushed
Tenderstem broccoli, blanched, to serve

For the cauliflower cream
1 large cauliflower (about 600g), cut into florets
250ml (1 cup) coconut cream
60ml (1/4 cup) filtered water
2 tbsp extra virgin coconut oil
1/2 tsp sea salt

1. Place the black pepper, allspice, cinnamon, nutmeg, coriander, cumin and cloves in a small bowl and mix to combine. Rub the spice mixture over the meat, rubbing well into the fatty bits. Really get your fingers into the meat, massaging it all over. Leave covered for at least 2 hours (or cover and refrigerate overnight for a stronger flavour).

2. Rub the oil into the meat, then sear in a hot frying pan until brown all over. Place in the slow cooker and add the bay leaves, stock, apple cider vinegar, passata and garlic. Cover and cook on low for 8 hours or high for 5 hours.

3. Take out the pork, place in a dish and use two forks to shred the meat. Put the shreds back in the slow cooker with the sauce and cook on high, uncovered, for 20 minutes, or until the sauce has thickened.

4. Meanwhile, make the cauliflower cream. Put the cauliflower, coconut cream, water, oil and salt in a large saucepan over a low heat. Cover and cook for 10 minutes, or until the cauliflower has softened, stirring occasionally to prevent burning (add an extra splash of water if needed). Blend with a stick blender (or use a potato masher) until smooth.

5. Divide the pork between serving bowls and serve with tenderstem broccoli and a dollop of cauliflower cream.

MASTER THE ART

ABUNDANCE BOWLS

The ingredients in each abundance bowl recipe are selected to be fantastic for fertility and incredibly delicious. Each bowl is nutritionally balanced and includes an abundance of colourful vegetables, good-quality protein and healthy fats to create harmony of taste, colour and nutritional benefit. All bowls are accompanied by a dressing, dip or sauce for a burst of flavour and are scattered with fresh herbs or sprouts.

Start with a vegetable base
(Half a plate or 3 cups)

Choose from:
- A rainbow of non-starchy vegetables (head to the veggie section on pages 184–199 for inspiration)

Layer on a palm-sized portion of protein

Choose from:
- Grass-fed meat
- Organic free-range poultry or eggs
- Wild-caught fish
- Organic legumes (ideally soaked before cooking, page 230)

Use healthy fats to cook your protein and flavour with herbs and spices

Add a dollop, drizzle or scatter with healthy fats
(1–2 tbsp)

Choose from:
- Avocado or avocado oil – try my Avocado and edamame smash (page 202)
- Coconut (desiccated, flakes, oil, yoghurt or cream)
- Dressing, sauce (pages 204–209) or Hummus (pages 200–201)
- Nuts (almonds, cashews, pecans, walnuts – you could make my Green dukkah on page 161)
- Seeds (hemp, pumpkin, sesame, sunflower)

Add a side portion of cooked starchy carbs
(2–3 tbsp or ½ cup)

Choose from:
- Root vegetables (beetroot, carrot, celeriac, parsnip, potato, squash, sweet potato)
- Organic legumes (ideally soaked before cooking)
- Organic whole grains or pseudo grains (buckwheat, quinoa, teff, brown or wild rice)

Finish with a sprinkling of concentrated nutrients
(1–2 tbsp)

Choose from:
- Fresh herbs
- Broccoli sprouts
- Citrus zest (unwaxed, lemon or lime)

Mexican abundance bowl

A filling, one-bowl wonder that delivers on taste. The Mexican-inspired flavours are deeply satisfying, and this is one of my favourites.

Serves 2

For the chicken

170g chipotle adobo Mexican chilli paste (see Pantry staples on page 85)
1 garlic clove, crushed
1 tbsp extra virgin olive oil
1 tsp honey
Sea salt and cracked black pepper
2 x 125g organic free-range chicken breasts

For the sweet potato

2 tsp olive oil
½ tsp Mexican chilli powder blend (see Pantry staples on page 91)
¼ tsp crushed chipotle chillies (see Pantry staples on page 85)
¼ tsp garlic powder
Sea salt
1 medium sweet potato, cubed

For the guacamole

1 tbsp horseradish root, finely grated (see Pantry staples on page 90)
1 ripe avocado, skin and stone removed
1 small red onion, finely chopped
Juice of ½ lime
Pinch of sea salt
½ bunch coriander leaves and stems, chopped

To serve

1 quantity of Mexican-style veggie rice (page 197)
Rocket
Coriander leaves, roughly chopped
Lime wedges

1. Preheat the oven to 180°C (350°F). Line two baking trays with plastic-free baking parchment.

2. First make the marinade for the chicken. Place the adobo paste, garlic, oil, honey, salt and black pepper in a medium bowl and whisk to combine. Add the chicken breasts and toss to coat. Set aside.

3. Next, prepare the sweet potato. Place the oil, Mexican chilli powder blend, chipotle chillies, garlic powder and a pinch of salt in a medium bowl and whisk to combine. Add the sweet potato and toss to coat.

4. Transfer the chicken and sweet potato to the prepared trays, ensuring the sweet potato is evenly spread. Bake for 20–25 minutes until the sweet potato is golden, the chicken is cooked through and the sauce has thickened.

5. Meanwhile, make the guacamole. Place all the ingredients in a food processor and process to a chunky consistency. Set aside.

6. Divide the veggie rice between two serving bowls, then layer up with the chicken and sweet potatoes. Serve with a big dollop of guacamole and a handful of rocket. Sprinkle with coriander and serve with lime wedges.

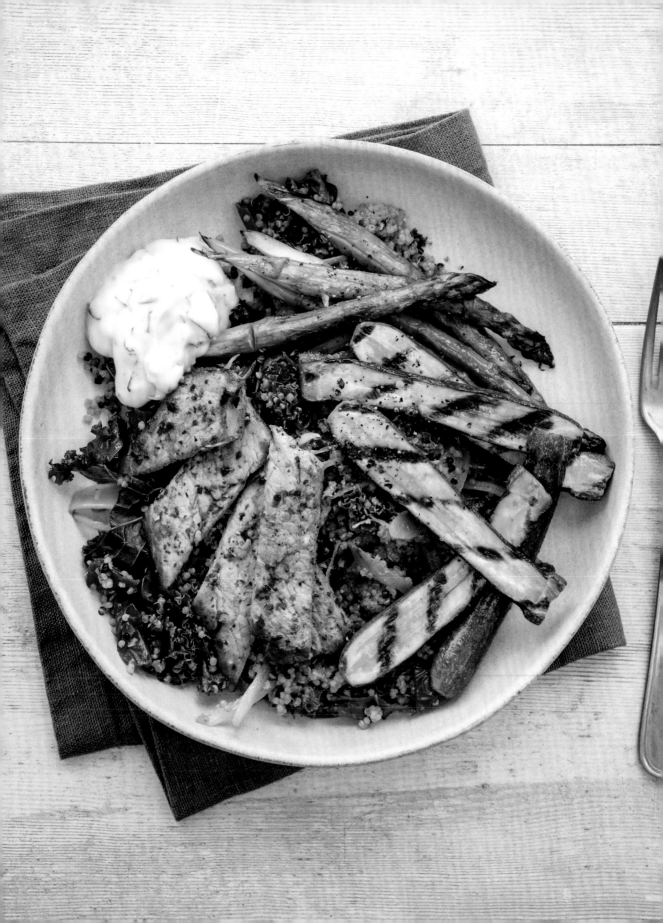

Mediterranean abundance bowl

A colourful dish inspired by Mediterranean flavours that delivers a healthy and tasty hit in one bowl and will leave you feeling wonderfully well fed.

Serves 2

For the garlic and lemon pork
1 tbsp olive oil
Zest of ½ lemon
½ tsp dried oregano
2 garlic cloves, crushed
2 x 120g free-range pork medallions

For the yoghurt dressing
125g (½ cup) coconut yoghurt

½ bunch (12g) flat-leaf parsley leaves, finely chopped

For the quinoa and kale tabbouleh
2 tsp olive oil
2 echalion shallots, sliced lengthways
Pinch of sea salt
120g (1 cup) cooked quinoa
30g (1 cup, tightly packed) kale leaves, finely chopped

6 sundried tomatoes, roughly chopped
Juice of ½ lemon

For the chargrilled spring veg
1 tbsp olive oil
Sea salt and cracked black pepper
6 asparagus spears, trimmed
6 baby courgettes, halved lengthways

1. First make the marinade for the pork. Place the oil, lemon zest, oregano and almost all the garlic in a shallow bowl and whisk to combine. Add the pork medallions, toss to coat and set aside in the fridge for at least 30 minutes to marinate.

2. While the pork is marinating make the yoghurt dressing. Place the yoghurt in a small bowl, add the parsley and remaining garlic and whisk to combine. Set aside.

3. Next make the tabbouleh. Heat the oil in a frying pan over a medium heat and fry the shallots and salt for 4–5 minutes, or until golden. Add the cooked quinoa and kale and cook for 1–2 minutes. Remove from the heat, add the sundried tomatoes, lemon juice and stir through. Set aside.

4. Place a griddle pan over a medium–high heat. Place the oil, a little salt and black pepper in a medium bowl, then add the asparagus and courgettes and toss to coat. Cook the pork medallions on the griddle for 10 minutes, turning to cook both sides, until the pork is cooked through. Add the vegetables to the griddle, turning to cooking both sides, for 5–6 minutes, or until tender.

5. To assemble, divide the quinoa tabbouleh between serving bowls, top with the chargrilled vegetables and pork. Add a spoonful of yoghurt dressing to serve.

Charlotte's notes

If you don't like pork, use chicken breasts.

Za'atar-baked aubergines *with* lemon tahini dressing

Herby, fresh and seedy, za'atar is one of my all-time favourite seasonings, and aubergines are the best vegetables for soaking up flavour. This fuss-free side is an easy and delicious way to bring more veg to your table.

Serves 2–4

4 tbsp extra virgin olive oil

1 tbsp za'atar

1 tbsp chopped lemon thyme, plus extra sprigs
  to serve

2 large aubergines, halved and scored in a
  diamond-shape pattern

Sea salt and cracked black pepper

½ quantity of Lemon tahini dressing
  (page 207), to serve

1 tbsp sesame seeds, to serve

1. Preheat the oven to 180°C (350°F). Line a baking tray with plastic-free baking parchment.

2. Place the oil, za'atar and chopped thyme in a small bowl and whisk to combine. Place the aubergine halves, cut-sides up, on the prepared baking tray. Sprinkle with salt and black pepper, brush with the infused oil and bake for 35–40 minutes, or until tender and golden.

3. While the aubergines are cooking, make the lemon tahini dressing. Set aside.

4. Place the aubergines on a serving plate and drizzle with the dressing. Scatter with the sesame seeds and sprigs of lemon thyme to serve.

Charlotte's notes

My favourite za'atar is by Steenbergs. They have a wonderful array of herbs and spices. You should also be able to find za'atar in the spices section of the supermarket.

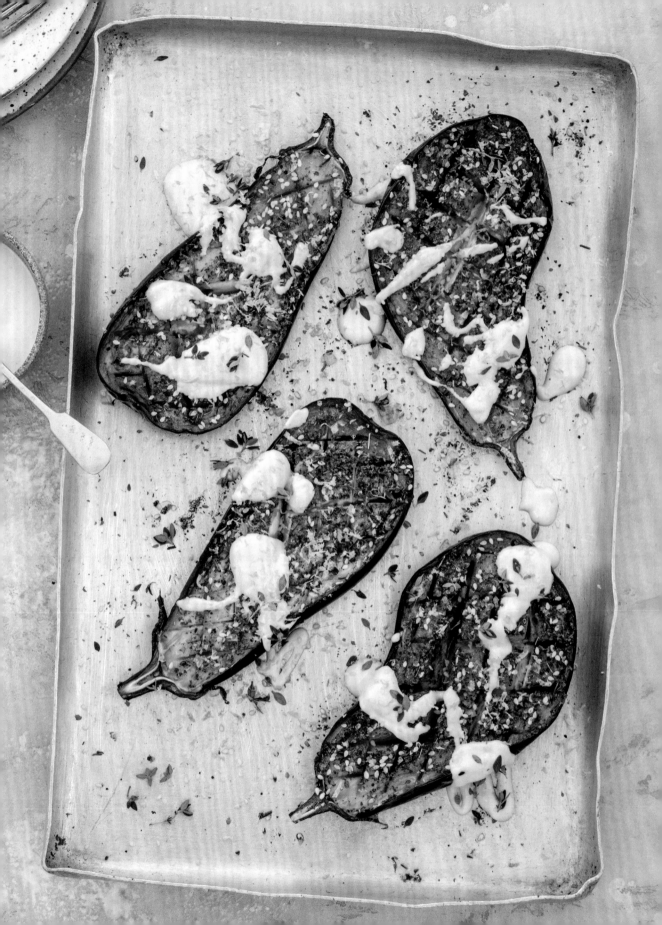

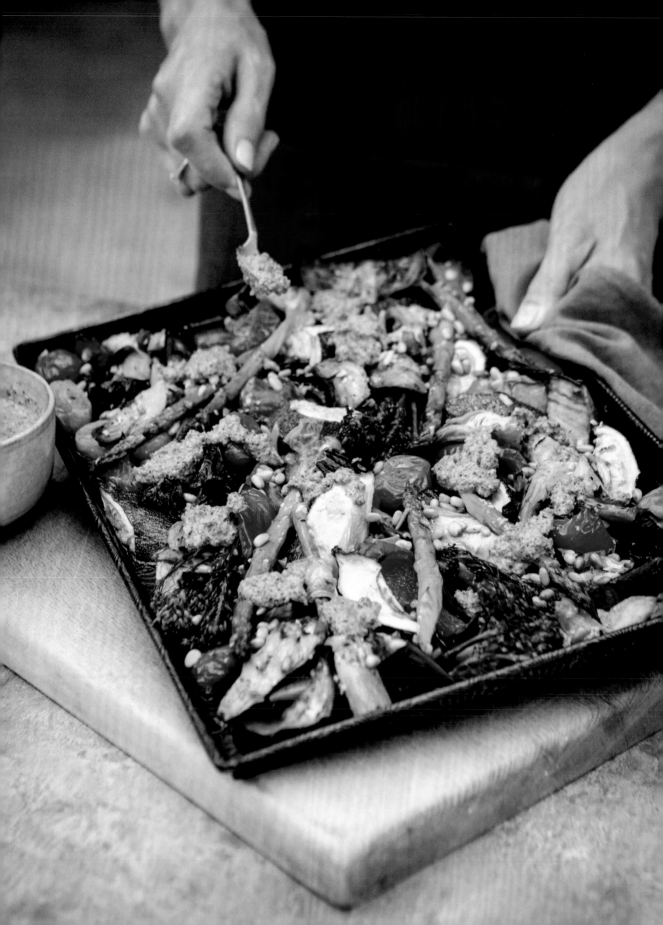

Summer vegetable traybake *with super-green walnut pesto*

This versatile summer veggie traybake is heaven on a plate – and just wait until you try the super-green pesto. Try adding poached eggs to make it into a simple supper.

Serves 4

1 red pepper, chopped into bite-sized chunks
1 small aubergine, chopped into bite-sized chunks
1 small courgette, chopped into bite-sized chunks
2 large garlic cloves, crushed
2 tbsp olive oil
Juice and zest of ½ lemon
Sea salt and cracked black pepper

14 mixed cherry tomatoes
190g jar chargrilled artichoke chunks, drained
12 asparagus tips (about 100g), trimmed
6 tenderstem broccoli stems (about 100g), trimmed
½ quantity of Super-green walnut pesto (page 202)
3 tbsp pine nuts, to serve

1. Preheat the oven to 180°C (350°f).

2. Place the red pepper, aubergine, courgette and garlic in a roasting tin. Drizzle with 1 tablespoon of the oil and the lemon juice, sprinkle with the lemon zest, season with salt and black pepper and toss to coat. Roast for 15 minutes.

3. Remove from the oven and scatter over the cherry tomatoes, artichoke chunks, asparagus tips and broccoli. Drizzle with the remaining oil, season and return to the oven for 15 minutes.

4. While the vegetables are in the oven, make the super-green walnut pesto. Set aside.

5. Divide the roasted vegetables between serving plates and drizzle with the pesto. Sprinkle with the pine nuts to serve.

Charlotte's notes

Leftover Super-green pesto can be used to make Green shakshuka (page 130) or to jazz up scrambled eggs (stir 1 teaspoon through eggs once scrambled).

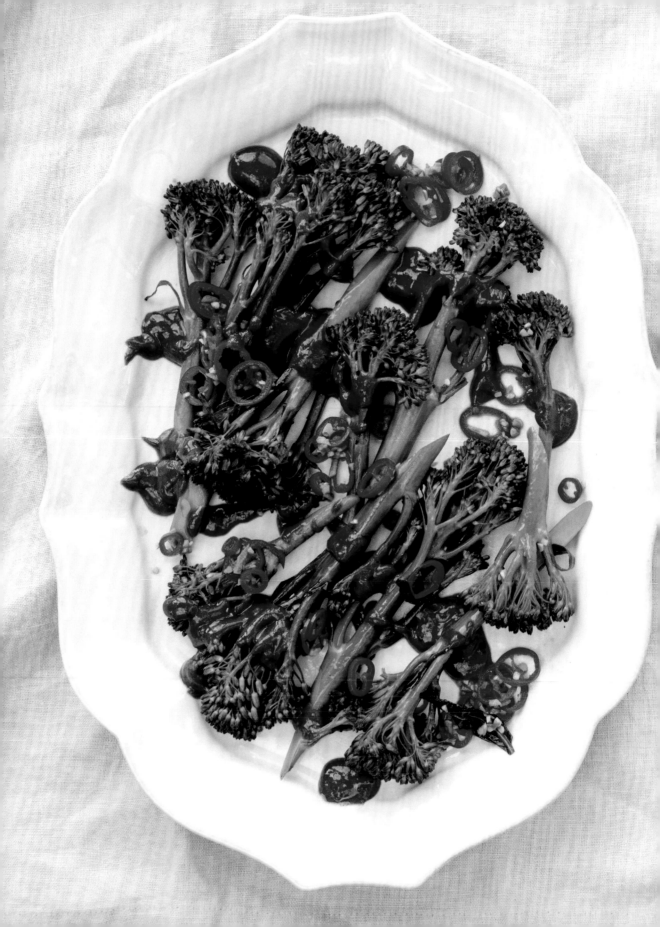

Garlic and chilli tenderstem *with*
Thai almond sauce

Bring more greens to the table with this spicy side dish. Big on flavour, this is an easy way to spruce up broccoli. This dish is perfect for sharing and combining with main courses.

Serves 2

1 tsp sesame oil
2 garlic cloves, crushed
1 red chilli, sliced
200g (12 stems) tenderstem broccoli, ends trimmed
1 tsp tamari or coconut aminos
Pinch of sea salt

For the Thai almond sauce
2 tbsp almond butter
2 tbsp tamari, or coconut aminos if avoiding soy (see Pantry staples on page 86)
Juice of 1 lime
¼ tsp chilli flakes

1. First make the Thai almond sauce. Place all the ingredients in a small bowl and whisk until smooth. Set aside.

2. Next, cook the broccoli. Place a frying pan over a medium heat. Add the oil, garlic and chilli and stir-fry for 1 minute until fragrant. Add the broccoli, tamari and salt and stir-fry for 2–3 minutes, or until the broccoli is vibrant.

3. Place the broccoli on a serving plate and drizzle with the almond sauce.

Charlotte's notes

• I love to serve this broccoli with Thai salmon cakes (page 151). As a side dish this serves two generously, but remember that vegetables should be front and centre of your plate.
• Leftover Thai almond sauce will keep in an airtight glass container in the fridge for up to three days. It's great served with stir-fried vegetables.

Curried cauliflower *with almonds*

Love, love, love! This curried cauliflower is such a winner. It goes well with salad or any protein. Why not create an Abundance bowl (pages 180–183) using this as your base?

Serves 2

1 tsp ground coriander
½ tsp ground cumin
½ tsp garam masala
¼ tsp turmeric
¼ tsp sea salt

1 tbsp extra virgin coconut oil
½ medium cauliflower
  (about 175g), cut into florets
30g (⅓ cup) flaked almonds

1. Preheat the oven to 180°C (350°F). Line a baking tray with plastic-free baking parchment.

2. Place the spices and salt in a small bowl and mix to combine. Melt the oil in a medium saucepan over a medium–high heat. Add the spices and cook for 1–2 minutes, or until fragrant. Add the cauliflower and toss to coat well.

3. Spread the cauliflower evenly on the prepared baking tray and roast for 20 minutes, turning halfway through cooking. Add the almonds, mix well and roast for a further 4–5 minutes, or until the almonds are golden-brown and the cauliflower is tender.

Charlotte's notes

Try making this into cauliflower rice: roast the cauliflower for 25 minutes, then grate in a food processor. Stir through the flaked almonds to serve.

Apple and black garlic sauerkraut

Sauerkraut is good for your gut and can be made easily at home. The green apple adds a delicious, sharper taste to this kraut and is balanced by the sweet, syrupy taste of black garlic. Serve with burgers (pages 177 and 178) or use it to jazz up a salad.

Fills a 750ml jar

1 organic white cabbage (about 850g), finely shredded
1 tbsp sea salt flakes
1 black garlic clove
1 green apple, peeled and diced

1. Place the cabbage in a large bowl, sprinkle with the salt and set aside for 5 minutes. Use a muddler or the end of a rolling pin to massage the cabbage until the juices start to escape.

2. Squeeze the black garlic out of its skin and mash with a fork. Add to the cabbage and use your hands to mix until well combined. Stir in the apple.

3. Transfer to a sterilised 750ml glass jar (see notes on page 192), pushing down firmly so that the cabbage is tightly packed with no gaps and the juices cover the top of the cabbage by 2cm (¾ inch). Top up with filtered water if needed, but leave at least 2cm (¾ inch) at the top of the jar for expansion.

4. Cover the jar with a clean tea towel or muslin cloth and secure with an elastic band. Place in a cool, dark place to start the fermentation process. Leave for 3–5 days, checking the fermentation every day to make sure the juices still completely cover the cabbage. Push the cabbage down and/or top up with filtered water if needed.

5. The sauerkraut is ready when bubbles start to appear on the surface. If you like a stronger flavour, you can leave the kraut at room temperature for another 2–3 days. Once you are happy with the flavour, remove the tea towel or muslin cloth, seal the jar with a lid and store in the fridge. The sauerkraut will keep for up to one month in the fridge.

White miso and turmeric kimchi

Make your own naturally fermented kimchi with cabbage, carrots and daikon in a tangy, spicy sauce.

Fills a 1 litre jar

1kg Chinese (napa) cabbage, cut into 2cm
   (³/4 inch) segments
85g sea salt
3 red chillies, deseeded and membranes
   removed, finely chopped
2.5cm (1 inch) piece of ginger, peeled
2.5cm (1 inch) piece of turmeric root, peeled

3 garlic cloves, peeled
2 tsp white miso paste
1½ tsp coconut sugar
3 tbsp filtered water
1 large carrot, coarsely grated
300g (2½ cups) daikon, coarsely grated
   (see notes)

1. Place the cabbage in a large bowl and rub in the salt. Allow to stand for 1 hour. Transfer the cabbage to a colander and rinse thoroughly. Allow to sit in the colander for 20 minutes to drain, then return to the bowl.

2. Place the chillies, ginger, turmeric, garlic, miso paste, coconut sugar and water in a blender and blend until smooth.

3. Add the carrot and daikon to the bowl with the cabbage and stir in the paste. Transfer to a 1-litre sterilised glass jar and press the mixture down to release any air bubbles and so that the juices completely cover the mixture. Leave about 2cm (¾ inch) of space at the top of the jar.

4. Cover the jar with a clean tea towel or muslin cloth and elastic band. Leave to ferment for 3–5 days in a cool, dark place. Check the fermentation every day to make sure the juices still completely cover the cabbage, pushing it down and/or topping up with filtered water if needed.

5. The kimchi is ready when bubbles start to appear on the surface. Test the flavour and leave for another 2–3 days if you like a stronger flavour. Once fermented to your desired level, seal the jar with a lid and store in the fridge. The kimchi will keep for up to one month in the fridge.

Charlotte's notes

• To sterilise a glass jar, preheat the oven to 120°C (250°F). Wash the jar in hot, soapy water, rinse and leave to dry, then place on a baking tray in the oven for 15 minutes.
• Daikon is a long, white, crunchy vegetable from the cabbage family and is also known as mooli.

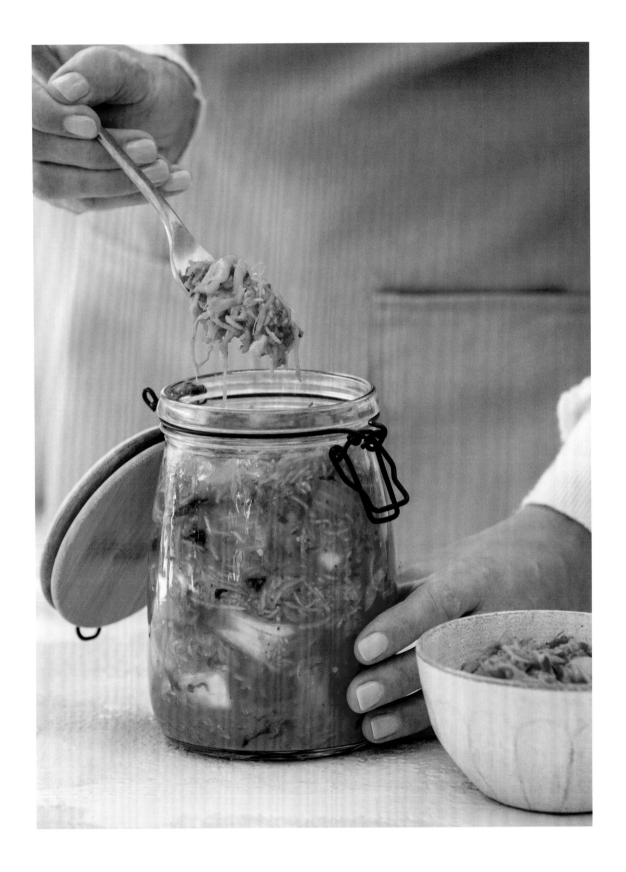

Veggie mash 3 ways

Looking for a nutrient-packed spin on classic mash? Choose from low-carb cheesy cauliflower, carotenoid-rich sweet potato or creamy celeriac.

Cheesy cauliflower

Serves 4

1 medium cauliflower (about 500g), cut into florets
80ml (⅓ cup) cashew milk (to make your own see page 137)
1 tbsp flavourless coconut oil
3 tbsp ground walnuts
1 tbsp nutritional yeast
Sea salt and cracked black pepper
1 tsp paprika

Steam the cauliflower over a saucepan of simmering water for 15–20 minutes, or until softened. Pour the water away, transfer the cauliflower to the saucepan and add the cashew milk, oil, ground walnuts, nutritional yeast, salt and black pepper. Blend until smooth using a hand-held stick blender. Sprinkle with the paprika to serve.

Sweet potato

Serves 4

2 medium sweet potatoes (about 450g), peeled and cut into 2.5cm (1 inch) dice
80ml (⅓ cup) cashew milk (to make your own see page 137)
1 tbsp flavourless coconut oil
Sea salt and cracked black pepper
¼–½ tsp ground cinnamon

Place the sweet potatoes in a saucepan, just cover with filtered water and bring to the boil. Reduce the heat and simmer for 10–12 minutes, or until soft and tender. Drain and return to the saucepan. Add the milk, oil, salt, black pepper and ¼ teaspoon of ground cinnamon. Blend until smooth using a hand-held stick blender or potato masher. Taste and add an extra ¼ teaspoon of cinnamon if desired.

Creamy celeriac

Serves 4

1 tbsp olive oil
1 small leek, white part only, finely sliced
Pinch of sea salt
1 small celeriac (about 400g), peeled and chopped into bite-sized chunks
125ml (½ cup) cashew milk (to make your own see page 137)
½ tsp Dijon mustard

Heat the oil in a medium saucepan over a medium heat. Add the leek and salt and cook for 3 minutes, or until soft. Add the celeriac and cashew milk, cover with a lid and cook for 15 minutes, or until the celeriac is tender. Remove from the heat and set aside to cool slightly. Add the mustard and blend until smooth using a hand-held stick blender or potato masher.

Veggie rice 3 ways

A perfect base for your protein of choice, veggie rice is an absolute nutrient powerhouse. Any excuse to get an extra helping of vegetables into a meal!

Thai-style egg-fried rice

Serves 4

2 tbsp extra virgin coconut oil

4 spring onions, finely sliced

1 (25g) bunch of coriander, stalks finely chopped, leaves roughly chopped

1 garlic clove, crushed

2.5cm (1 inch) piece of ginger, peeled and finely grated

1 red chilli, seeds and membranes removed, finely chopped

1 medium cauliflower (about 500g), grated

2 stalks of kale, stems removed and leaves shredded

1 tbsp Thai spice seasoning (see Pantry staples on page 93)

2 large organic free-range eggs, beaten (optional)

1 tbsp tamari or coconut aminos if avoiding soy (see Pantry staples on page 86)

4 tbsp cashews, toasted and roughly chopped

Heat 1 tablespoon of the oil in a large frying pan over a medium heat. Add the spring onions, coriander stalks, garlic, ginger and chilli and cook for 1–2 minutes, or until fragrant. Add the cauliflower and kale and stir in the Thai spice seasoning and the remaining oil. Mix well to combine. Create a well in the centre, add the beaten eggs (if using) and tamari (or coconut aminos) and stir-fry until the eggs are cooked and the cauliflower is golden. Serve the rice in bowls and top with the cashews and coriander leaves to serve.

Charlotte's notes

- Make life easier and use a food processor to grate the cauliflower.
- If you include the eggs, this rice dish makes a perfect light lunch; leave them out if you're serving it with another protein source.
- Use broccoli instead of cauliflower for extra green goodness!

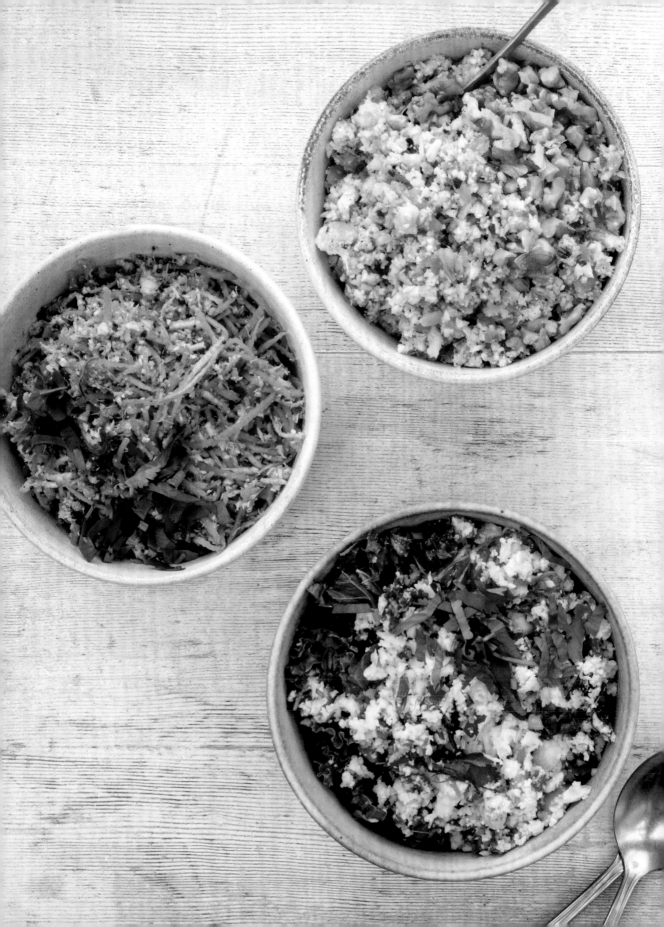

Indian style

Serves 4

1 tbsp olive oil
1 onion, finely diced
1 garlic clove, crushed
1 bunch (25g) coriander, stalks finely chopped,
   leaves roughly chopped
¼ tsp sea salt
1 tbsp tsp pilau seasoning blend
   (see Pantry staples on page 92)
1 medium cauliflower (about 500g), grated
2 tbsp chopped walnuts

Heat the oil in a large frying pan over a
medium heat. Add the onion, garlic,
coriander stalks and salt and cook for 3–4
minutes, or until the onion is beginning to
soften. Add the pilau seasoning blend and
cauliflower, mix well and cook for 5 minutes,
or until lightly golden. Stir through the
walnuts and coriander leaves to serve.

Mexican style

Serves 4

½ head of broccoli (about 250g), grated
½ head of cauliflower (about 250g), grated
1 carrot, finely grated
1 tbsp Mexican chilli powder blend
   (see Pantry staples in page 91)
Sea salt and cracked black pepper
1 tbsp olive oil
1 garlic clove, crushed
1 bunch (25g) coriander, stalks finely chopped,
   leaves roughly chopped
Juice of ½ lime

Place the broccoli, cauliflower and carrot in
a medium bowl and toss with the Mexican
chilli powder blend, salt and black pepper.
Heat the oil in a frying pan over a medium
heat, add the garlic and coriander stalks and
gently fry for 1 minute, or until fragrant. Add
the grated broccoli and cauliflower and
warm through, then stir in the coriander
leaves and lime juice to serve.

Veggie crisps

A healthy-eating game changer – ditch processed crisps for these healthy veggie alternatives. Delicious served with homemade Hummus (pages 200–201).

Sesame-coated sweet potato crisps

Serves 2

2 medium sweet potatoes (about 450g), scrubbed and sliced very thinly and evenly (use a mandolin if you have one)
2–3 tbsp olive oil
2 tbsp mixed black and white sesame seeds (see Pantry staples on page 93)
¼ tsp ground cinnamon (optional)
Sea salt flakes

1. Preheat the oven to 150°C (300°F). Line a large baking tray with plastic-free baking parchment.

2. Place the sweet potato slices in a large bowl, drizzle with the olive oil and toss to coat, using your hands. Spread the slices over the prepared baking tray in a single layer. Sprinkle over the sesame seeds, cinnamon (if using) and salt.

3. Bake for 20–25 minutes, or until golden and crisp. Keep a close eye on them as they can go from perfect to burnt very quickly. Remove from the oven and leave to cool for 5 minutes before serving.

Cheesy kale crisps

Serves 2

150g (5 cups) kale leaves, stalks removed and leaves torn
1 tbsp olive oil
Garlic salt
1 tbsp nutritional yeast flakes (see Pantry staples on page 91)
½ tsp chilli flakes (optional)

1. Preheat the oven to 150°C (300°F). Line a large baking tray with plastic-free baking parchment.

2. Place the kale in a large bowl and drizzle with the oil. Season well with garlic salt and sprinkle over the nutritional yeast and chilli flakes (if using). Gently mix with your hands to make sure all the leaves are well coated.

3. Spread the kale leaves evenly over the prepared tray and bake for 10–12 minutes, or until crisp. Keep a close eye on them as they can burn easily. Remove from the oven and leave to cool completely. They will crisp up on cooling.

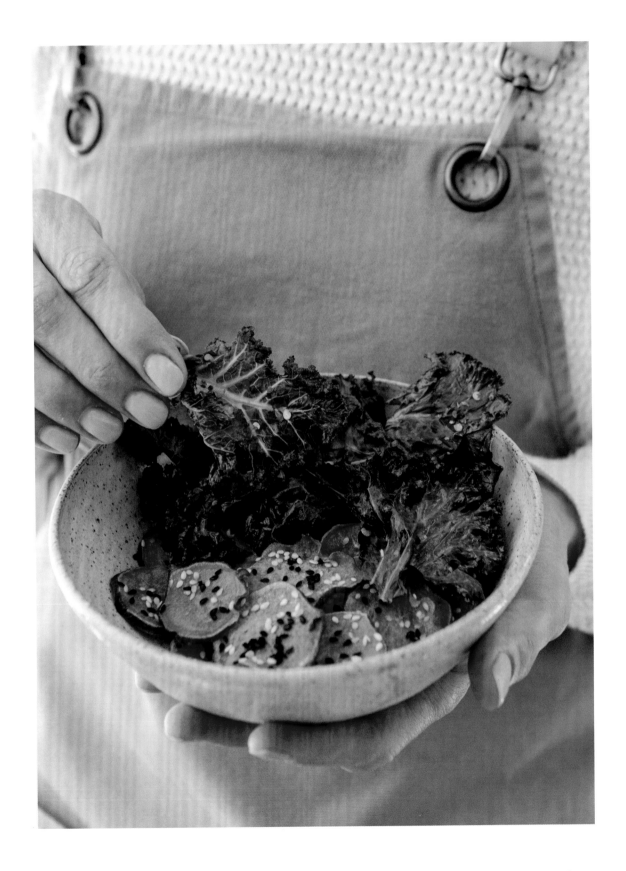

Hummus 3 ways

Hummus is a total crowd pleaser and one of my fridge staples. I've created three flavours, including two chickpea-free options. There's nothing wrong with chickpeas, but some people struggle to digest them, so these are great alternatives. Try spreading hummus on a slice of Seed and nut gluten-free loaf (page 136), serving with homemade Veggie crisps (page 198) or Super-seedy crackers (page 146).

Roasted beetroot and rosemary

Makes 310g (1½ cups)

5 medium beetroot, quartered
1 large garlic clove
1 tbsp olive oil, plus extra for drizzling
½ tsp sea salt
1 rosemary sprig, leaves stripped
   and chopped
3 tbsp light (hulled) tahini
½ tsp ground cumin
¼ tsp mild chilli powder (optional)
Juice of ½ lemon
1–2 tbsp filtered water

Preheat the oven to 180°C (350°F). Line a small baking tray with plastic-free baking parchment. Place the beetroot and garlic on the prepared tray and drizzle with the oil. Sprinkle with the salt and rosemary and roast for 45–60 minutes, or until tender. Set aside to cool, then transfer to a food processor. Add the tahini, cumin, chilli powder (if using), lemon juice and 1 tablespoon of water. Process until smooth, adding an extra tablespoon of water to thin if desired. Drizzle with extra oil to serve.

Pea and mint

Makes 430g (2 cups)

1 x 350g jar chickpeas, drained and rinsed
125g (1 cup) frozen peas, thawed slightly
1 tbsp light (hulled) tahini
1 small garlic clove, crushed
Juice of 1 lemon
2 tbsp extra virgin olive oil,
   plus extra for drizzling
1 tbsp chopped mint leaves,
   plus extra to serve
Sea salt and cracked black pepper
1 tbsp filtered water

Place the chickpeas, peas, tahini, garlic, lemon juice, oil, mint, salt and black pepper in a food processor and process until smooth. Add the water to thin, if desired. Drizzle with extra oil and sprinkle with chopped mint to serve.

Roasted carrot and turmeric

Makes 300g (1½ cups)

6 large carrots, peeled and cut into chunks
1 large garlic clove
½ tsp sea salt
2 tbsp olive oil, plus extra for drizzling
3 tbsp light (hulled) tahini
½ tsp mild curry powder
½ tsp turmeric
Juice of ½ lemon
1–2 tbsp filtered water
½ tsp each of black and white sesame seeds,
   for sprinkling

Preheat the oven to 180°C (350°F). Line a
small baking tray with plastic-free baking
parchment. Place the carrots and garlic on
the prepared tray. Sprinkle with the salt and
drizzle with 1 tablespoon of the oil. Roast
for 35–40 minutes, or until tender. Set aside
to cool, then transfer to a food processor.
Add the remaining oil, tahini, curry powder,
turmeric, lemon juice and 1 tablespoon of
water. Process until smooth, adding an
extra tablespoon of water to thin if desired.
Drizzle with extra oil and sprinkle with the
sesame seeds to serve.

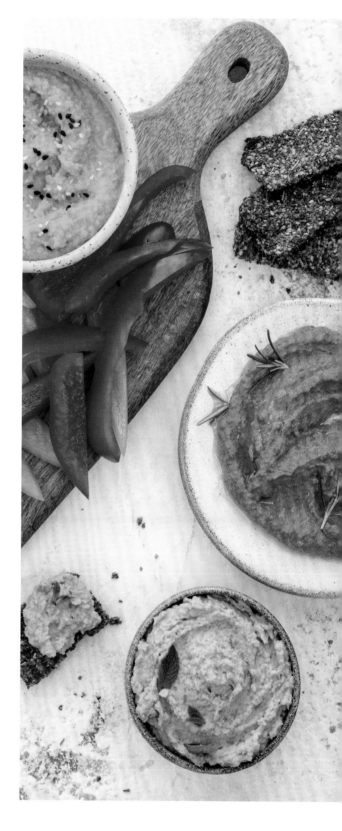

Avocado and edamame smash

Serve this smash with burgers (pages 177 and 178) or spread on toasted slices of Seed and nut loaf (page 136) for avo toast.

Makes 300g (1½ cups)

140g (1 cup) frozen shelled edamame, thawed
1 avocado, skin and stone removed
1 tbsp finely grated horseradish root
   (see notes)
½ small red onion, finely chopped
1 garlic clove, crushed
1 tbsp lime juice
¼ tsp sea salt
1 tbsp chopped coriander

Place half the edamame beans and the avocado in a medium bowl and roughly mash with a fork. Add the remaining edamame beans, horseradish, red onion, garlic, lime juice, salt and coriander and mix to combine.

Charlotte's notes

• Find fresh horseradish root next to fresh ginger and garlic in the supermarket.

Super-green walnut pesto

Use this fresh zingy pesto to drizzle over a Summer vegetable traybake (page 187), to make Green shakshuka (page 130) or simply to jazz up scrambled eggs.

Makes 330g (1½ cups)

35g (¼ cup) pistachios
30g (¼ cup) walnuts
2 large handfuls each of basil, rocket and kale
2 large garlic cloves, peeled and crushed
Juice and zest of 1 lemon
3 tbsp nutritional yeast (see Pantry staples
   on page 91)
½ tsp sea salt
¼ tsp cracked black pepper
6 tbsp extra virgin olive oil

Place the pistachios and walnuts in a food processor and process until roughly chopped. Add the basil, rocket, kale, garlic, lemon juice and zest, nutritional yeast, salt and pepper and process to finely chop. Scrape down the sides, then with the machine running, slowly add the oil. If the pesto is too thick, thin it out with a few tablespoons of filtered water.

Charlotte's notes

• For a nut-free pesto, use sunflower and pumpkin seeds instead of walnuts.
• Stir 1 teaspoon of pesto through scrambled eggs for a simple but delicious meal.
• Pesto will keep in an airtight glass container in the fridge for up to one week.

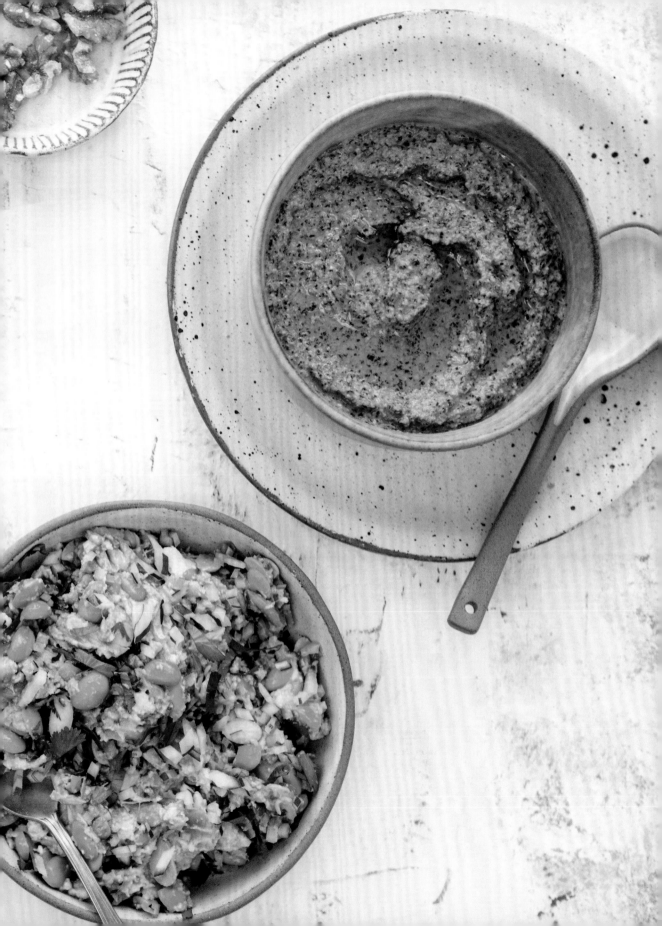

Dressings

Dressings are a great way to add flavour and extra nutrition to your meals. Here are a variety of my favourites to suit a range of cuisines.

Yoghurt lemon dressing

Makes 80ml (⅓ cup)

2 tbsp coconut yoghurt
Juice and zest of 1 lemon
1 tbsp olive oil
½ tsp honey
1 garlic clove, crushed
Sea salt and cracked black pepper

Place the coconut yoghurt, lemon juice, olive oil, honey, garlic, water, salt and pepper in a small bowl and whisk until smooth and creamy. Stir in the lemon zest.

Creamy cashew dressing

Makes 125 ml (½ cup)

90g (⅓ cup) smooth cashew butter
60ml (¼ cup) warm filtered water
Juice of 1 lemon
2 tsp extra virgin olive oil
1 small garlic clove, crushed
¼ tsp onion powder
¼ tsp sea salt
Pinch of cracked black pepper
½ tsp dried parsley
½ tsp dried dill

Place the cashew butter, water, lemon juice, oil, garlic, onion powder, salt and black pepper in a high-speed blender and blend until smooth. Remove from the blender and gently stir in the dried herbs.

Chilli lime dressing

Makes 125ml (½ cup)

125g (½ cup) coconut yoghurt
Juice of 1 lime
1 small red chilli, deseeded and finely chopped
Pinch of sea salt

Place the coconut yoghurt, lime juice, red chilli and salt in a small bowl and whisk until smooth.

Green goddess dressing

Makes 310 ml (1¼ cups)

1 avocado
85g (⅓ cup) coconut yoghurt
Juice of 1 lemon
1 garlic clove, crushed
Handful each of fresh chives, coriander
    and parsley
Sea salt and cracked black pepper
4–5 tbsp olive oil

Place the avocado, coconut yoghurt, lemon juice, garlic, herbs, salt and black pepper in a food processor and process until the herbs are finely chopped and the ingredients are well combined. With the machine running, slowly add the olive oil until the dressing is smooth and creamy.

Caesar dressing

Makes 125 ml (½ cup)

70g (¼ cup) cashew butter
Juice of ½ lemon
1½ tsp Dijon mustard
1½ tsp tamari
1 tbsp extra virgin olive oil
1 garlic clove, crushed
1½ tsp nutritional yeast (see Pantry
    staples on page 91)
1 tsp balsamic vinegar
2 tbsp warm filtered water

Place the cashew butter, lemon juice, mustard, tamari, olive oil, garlic, nutritional yeast, balsamic vinegar and water in a small food processor or blender and process until completely smooth.

Lemon mustard dressing

Makes 60 ml (¼ cup)

Juice of ½ large lemon
1½ tbsp extra virgin olive oil
¾ tsp Dijon mustard
¼ tsp raw honey
Sea salt and cracked black pepper

Place the lemon juice, olive oil, mustard, honey, salt and pepper in a small bowl and whisk until smooth.

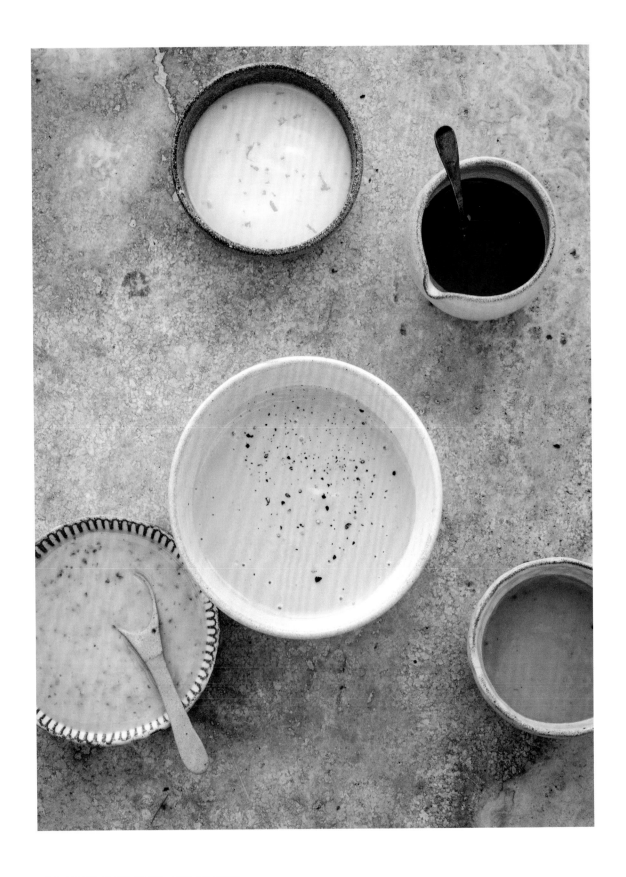

Spicy cashew dressing

Makes 125 ml (½ cup)

90g (⅓ cup) smooth cashew butter
60ml (¼ cup) warm filtered water
Juice of 1 lemon
2 tsp extra virgin olive oil
1 small garlic clove, crushed
1 tsp smoked sriracha chilli sauce
   (see Pantry staples on page 93)
¼ tsp onion powder
¼ tsp sea salt
Pinch of cracked black pepper

Place the cashew butter, water, lemon juice, olive oil, garlic, sriracha, onion powder, salt and black pepper in a small food processor and process until smooth.

Miso ginger dressing

Makes 125 ml (½ cup)

80g (¼ cup) white miso paste
2 tsp grated ginger
2 tsp raw honey
1 tbsp sesame oil
80ml (⅓ cup) warm filtered water

Place the miso paste, ginger, honey, sesame oil and water in a small food processor and process until smooth.

Lemon tahini dressing

Makes 310 ml (1¼ cups)

130g (½ cup) light (hulled) tahini
Juice and zest of 1 large lemon
2 tbsp apple cider vinegar
1 tbsp extra virgin olive oil
1 garlic clove, crushed
½ tsp sea salt
60–125ml (¼–½ cup) filtered water

Place the tahini, lemon juice and zest, apple cider vinegar, olive oil, garlic, salt and 60ml (¼ cup) of water in a small food processor and process until smooth and creamy. With the machine running, add extra water, 1 tablespoon at a time, until the dressing reaches a pourable consistency.

Charlotte's notes

Use light (hulled) tahini in this dressing as the seeds have been hulled and the flavour is less bitter.

Sauces

These sauces will add bags of flavour to many recipes. Serve Cashew ginger sauce with courgette noodles (page 142), swirl Salsa verde through soup (page 144) or use it as a pizza topping (page 174). Failproof tomato sauce can be used for recipes that call for chopped tomatoes or passata or use No-mato sauce if you don't like tomatoes or are avoiding nightshades!

Cashew ginger sauce

Makes 180ml (¾ cup)

4 tbsp smooth cashew butter
1 tbsp ginger, peeled and grated
1 garlic clove, crushed
3 tbsp tamari, or coconut aminos if avoiding
  soy (see Pantry staples on page 86)
Juice of ½ lemon
1 tsp raw honey
90ml (⅓ cup) warm filtered water

Place the cashew butter, ginger, garlic, tamari, lemon juice, honey and water in a jug and use a stick blender (or whisk) to blend until smooth.

Charlotte's notes

• You can use frozen chopped ginger for ease.
• For a nut-free version, swap the cashew butter for tahini.

Failproof tomato sauce

Makes 1.5l (6 cups)

2 tbsp olive oil
1 medium onion, finely diced
2 celery stalks, finely chopped
2 medium carrots, finely chopped
3 garlic cloves, crushed
Sea salt and cracked black pepper
2 tbsp tomato purée
2 x 680g jars passata rustica
Handful each of basil and parsley leaves,
  roughly chopped (optional, omit for use
  in curries)

1. Heat the oil in a large saucepan over a medium heat. Add the onion, celery, carrots, garlic, salt and black pepper and cook, stirring frequently, for 10 minutes, or until the vegetables have softened.

2. Stir in the tomato purée, passata and herbs (if using) and bring to a boil, then reduce the heat and simmer for 30 minutes.

3. Use a stick blender to blend to your desired consistency. For a chunky, more rustic sauce, blend for a shorter time; if you prefer a smooth sauce, blend for a little longer.

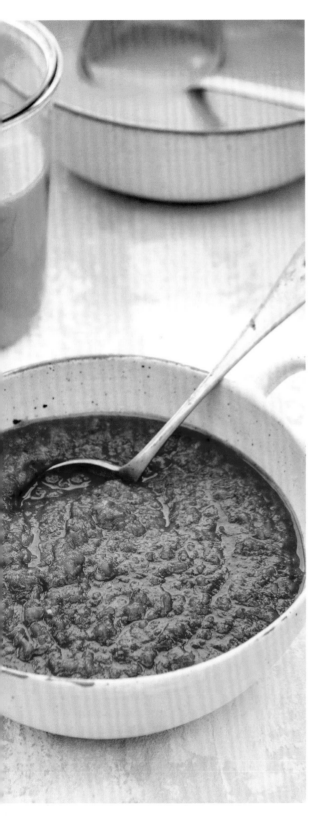

No-mato sauce

Makes 1.5l (6 cups)

2 tbsp olive oil
12 medium carrots, peeled and chopped
1 tsp sea salt
¼ tsp onion powder
625ml (2½ cups) vegetable stock
  (to make you own, see page 152)
2 tbsp tamari, or coconut aminos if avoiding soy
  (see Pantry staples on page 86)

1. Heat the oil in a large saucepan over a medium heat. Add the carrots, salt and onion powder and sauté for 3–4 minutes, or until the carrots begin to soften.

2. Add the stock and bring to a boil. Reduce the heat to low and simmer, covered, for 10 minutes, or until the carrots are tender. Transfer to a blender, add the tamari and blend until smooth.

Salsa verde

Makes 180 ml (¾ cup)

1 bunch (25g) flat-leaf parsley
1 bunch (25g) basil
½ bunch (12g) chives, chopped
2 tsp capers
2 garlic cloves, crushed
2 tbsp sherry vinegar (see Pantry
  staples on page 94)
4 tbsp extra virgin olive oil
Sea salt and cracked black pepper

Place the parsley, basil, chives, capers, garlic, sherry vinegar, olive oil, salt and pepper in a small food processor and blend to a chunky consistency.

POWER BARS

These no-bake power bars are bursting with all the good things and are simple to make. High in fibre, healthy fats and protein, they will give you a burst of energy.

The formula

Base ingredients

- 70g (⅓ cup) coconut oil (flavourless or extra virgin)
- 10 medjool dates, pitted
- 125g (1¼ cups) gluten-free rolled oats
- 35g (¼ cup) sunflower seeds
- 20g (⅛ cup) pumpkin seeds

Binding ingredients

- 60g (¼ cup) nut or seed butter of choice

Flavourings

3 tbsp:
- Ground nuts, cacao powder, desiccated coconut

+

2 tbsp:
- Dried fruit (unsweetened and unsulphured) or cacao nibs

Extract

¼ tsp:
- Almond
- Lemon
- Orange
- Peppermint
- Vanilla

Makes 24 squares

Cherry Bakewell

70g (⅓ cup) flavourless coconut oil
10 medjool dates, pitted
125g (1¼ cups) gluten-free rolled oats
35g (¼ cup) sunflower seeds
20g (⅛ cup) pumpkin seeds
3 tbsp ground almonds
2 tbsp tart cherries (unsweetened and
    unsulphured)
60g (¼ cup) smooth almond butter
¼ tsp pure almond extract

Mint chocolate

70g (⅓ cup) flavourless coconut oil
10 medjool dates, pitted
125g (1¼ cups) gluten-free rolled oats
35g (¼ cup) sunflower seeds
20g (⅛ cup) pumpkin seeds
3 tbsp raw cacao powder
2 tbsp cacao nibs
60g (¼ cup) smooth cashew butter
¼ tsp pure peppermint extract

Tropical

70g (⅓ cup) extra virgin coconut oil
10 medjool dates, pitted
125g (1¼ cups) gluten-free rolled oats
35g (¼ cup) sunflower seeds
20g (⅛ cup) pumpkin seeds
3 tbsp desiccated coconut
2 tbsp dried pineapple (unsweetened
    and unsulphured, see notes)
60g (¼ cup) smooth cashew butter
¼ tsp pure vanilla extract

1. Line a lightly greased 15 x 20cm
(6 x 8 inch) tin with plastic-free baking
parchment.

2. Melt the oil in a small saucepan over a
low heat, then pour into a food processor.
Add the remaining ingredients and process
until well combined.

3. Press the mixture into the prepared tin
and place in the freezer for 30–40 minutes,
or until firm. Cut into squares and serve.

Charlotte's notes

• For the tropical bars, look for gently baked
pineapple with nothing added (no
sweeteners) and unsulphured. I like the
brand Urban Fruit.
• You can store the bars in an airtight glass
container in the fridge for up to two weeks.

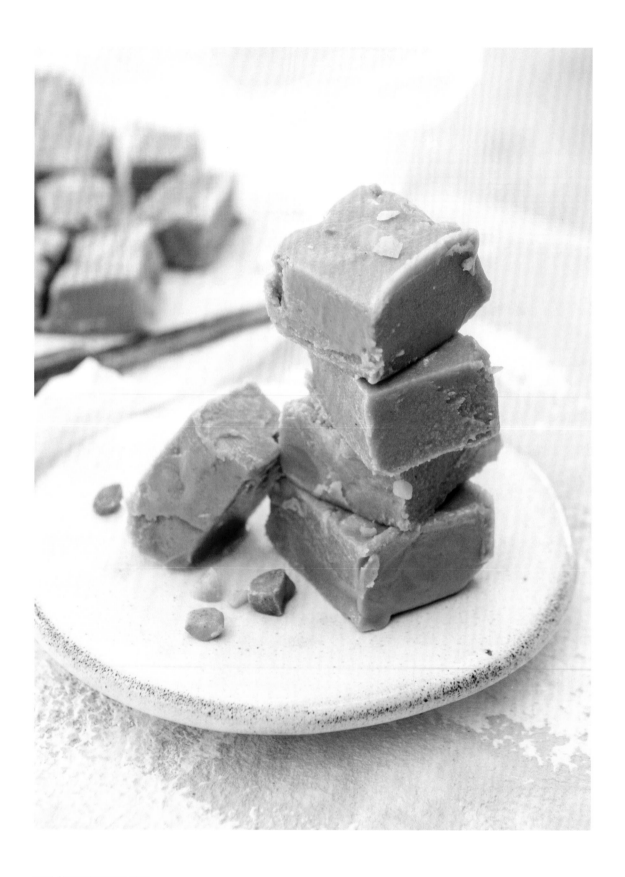

Salted macadamia and cashew butter fudge

This recipe delivers the perfect balance of salty-sweet, melt-in-the-mouth fudginess in every bite.

Makes 28 squares

210g (³/4 cup) smooth cashew butter
70g (¼ cup) smooth macadamia butter
160ml (²/3 cup) extra virgin coconut oil, plus
   extra for greasing
85g (¼ cup) honey

1 tsp pure vanilla extract
½ tsp fine sea salt
3 tbsp lightly toasted macadamia nuts,
   roughly chopped

1. Grease a 15 x 20cm (6 x 8 inch) baking tin with coconut oil and line with plastic-free baking parchment.

2. Place the cashew butter, macadamia butter, coconut oil, honey, vanilla extract and salt in a medium saucepan over a low heat, whisking until melted and well combined.

3. Remove from the heat and stir in 2 tablespoons of the macadamia nuts. Pour into the prepared tin, sprinkle with the remaining macadamia nuts and place in the fridge for at least 4 hours or overnight.

4. Remove from the fridge, turn out and slice into 28 squares. Refrigerate until ready to eat.

Charlotte's notes

• If you don't have macadamia nut butter, use 280g (1 cup) cashew butter instead. You could also try almond butter.
• The fudge melts quickly at room temperature. Store in an airtight glass container in the fridge for up to two weeks or keep in the freezer for up to one month (transfer a piece to the fridge to thaw before eating). I recommend lining your container and separating each fudge layer with plastic-free baking parchment to stop it clumping together.

Dreamy chocolate tahini brownies

These dreamy brownies are packed with rich chocolate and smooth tahini. They're made from just a few ingredients and taste utterly delicious.

Makes 16 squares

30g (1/4 cup) ground almonds
40g (1/3 cup) raw cacao powder, sifted
1 tsp baking powder
1/4 tsp bicarbonate of soda
1/4 tsp fine sea salt
50g (1/4 cup) flavourless coconut oil
100g (3/4 cup) dark chocolate (90% cocoa solids), roughly chopped

85g (1/3 cup) light (hulled) tahini
170g (1/2 cup) honey
2 tsp pure vanilla extract
2 large organic free-range eggs
Flaked sea salt

1. Preheat the oven to 160°C (325°F). Grease and line a 20cm (8 inch) square tin with plastic-free baking parchment.

2. Place the ground almonds, cacao powder, baking powder, bicarbonate of soda and salt in a medium bowl and mix to combine.

3. Place the oil and 70g (1/2 cup) of the chocolate in a medium heatproof bowl over a saucepan of gently simmering water (the bowl shouldn't touch the water) and stir for 2–3 minutes, or until smooth. Set aside to cool.

4. Place the tahini, honey, vanilla and eggs in a large bowl and whisk to combine. Add the cooled chocolate mixture and whisk until smooth. Add the flour mixture and fold to combine.

5. Pour the mixture into the prepared tin and sprinkle with the remaining 30g (1/4 cup) of chocolate and a little flaked salt. Bake for 30–35 minutes, or until set and when a skewer inserted into the centre comes out clean. Allow to cool completely, then remove from the tin and cut into 16 squares.

MASTER THE ART

FAT BOMBS

Fat bombs are so called because they are loaded with fat-rich ingredients. These low-carbohydrate treats fill you up fast and satisfy sweet cravings. If you usually fancy something sweet after a meal, try one of these beauties instead.

The formula

Base ingredients

- 100g coconut oil (extra virgin or flavourless)

+

- 130g nut butter of your choice

Optional sweetener (try without!)

- ½–1 tsp honey, date syrup, coconut syrup or maple syrup

Flavourings

- ¼ –1½ tsp extract* (almond, lemon, orange, peppermint, vanilla), miso paste, cacao powder, matcha powder, ground cinnamon or other spices of your choice

*Extracts are bold flavours, so less is more (start with ¼ tsp)

Makes 36 bombs

Almond cinnamon

100g (½ cup) extra virgin coconut oil
130g (½ cup) smooth almond butter
1 tsp honey (optional)
1 tsp pure vanilla extract
½ tsp ground cinnamon, sifted

Miso salted cashew

100g (½ cup) flavourless coconut oil
130g (½ cup) smooth cashew butter
1 tsp pure maple syrup (optional)
1 tsp white miso paste
¼ tsp sea salt

Pistachio chocolate orange

100g (½ cup) extra virgin coconut oil
130g (½ cup) smooth pistachio butter
1 tsp honey (optional)
¼ tsp pure orange extract
1½ tsp cacao powder, sifted

1. Place the oil, nut butter and sweetener (if using) in a small saucepan over a low heat and cook, stirring continuously, until melted and well combined. Add the flavourings and whisk until smooth.

2. Pour the mixture into silicone mini cup moulds and place on a baking tray in the freezer for 30–60 minutes, or until firm. Remove from the moulds and store in an airtight glass container in the fridge.

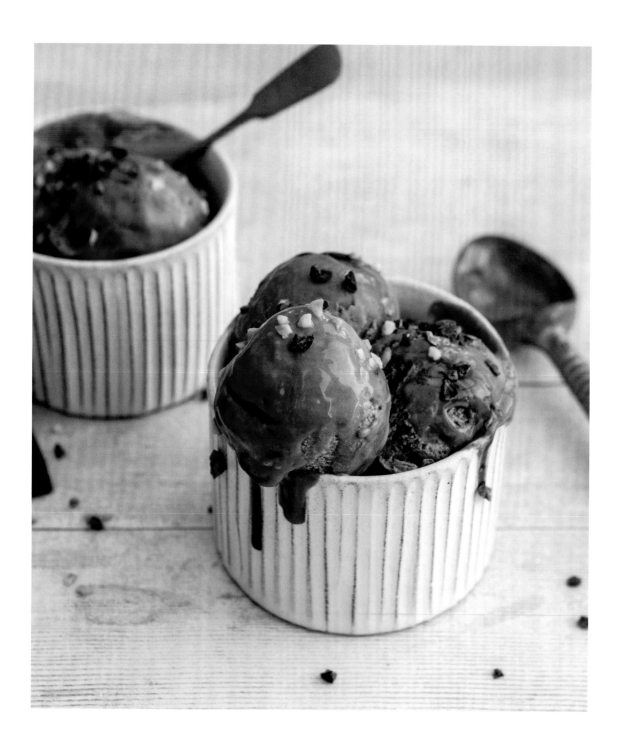

Chocolate-hazelnut n'ice cream

Creamy chocolate ice cream classically paired with hazelnut – it's simple and delicious. If you are not familiar with frozen banana ice cream yet, you are going to love it! Simply blend frozen bananas until smooth and you have a deliciously creamy 'n'ice' cream.

Serves 2

2 frozen bananas

3 tbsp cacao powder, sifted

2 heaped tbsp hazelnut butter

1–2 tbsp hazelnut milk (to make your own, see page 137)

2 tbsp roasted chopped hazelnuts, plus extra for sprinkling

1 tbsp pure maple syrup

1 tsp pure vanilla extract

4 squares (60g) dark chocolate (90% cocoa solids), roughly chopped

Cacao nibs, for sprinkling (see Pantry staples on page 85)

1. Place the bananas, cacao powder, hazelnut butter and 1 tablespoon of the hazelnut milk in a high-speed blender and blend until smooth. This can take a while and you may need to stop frequently to mix the ingredients and push down with your blender's tamper to achieve the perfect texture and consistency. Add an extra tablespoon of milk to thin if needed (try not to add any more than this as it can make the finished ice cream grainy with small ice crystals).

2. Transfer the ice cream mixture into a glass freezer-safe container, add the chopped hazelnuts, maple syrup, vanilla extract and chocolate and stir gently to combine.

3. Freeze for 3 hours, mixing well every 30 minutes. (Don't be tempted to skip the mixing step – this prevents ice crystals forming). After 3 hours, serve immediately, scooped into bowls and sprinkled with extra chopped hazelnuts and cacao nibs.

Charlotte's notes

- If you leave the ice cream to freeze for longer than 3 hours, remove from the freezer and let thaw for 30 minutes before serving as the ice cream will be solid.
- To obtain a perfect scoop, dip your ice cream scoop into hot water before use.
- Store ice cream in an airtight glass container in the freezer for up to one week.

Antioxidant burst soft serve

Perfect for a hot day, this soft serve is crammed with antioxidants.

Serves 2

70g (½ cup) frozen wild blueberries
70g (½ cup) frozen mango, thawed slightly
½ frozen banana, thawed slightly
½ frozen avocado, thawed slightly
1 tbsp coconut yoghurt

1 tsp wild blueberry powder
 (see Pantry staples on page 94)
60–125ml (¼–½ cup) coconut milk
 (to make your own, see page 137)
2 tbsp pistachios, finely chopped, to serve

1. Place the blueberries, mango, banana, avocado, coconut yoghurt, blueberry powder and 60ml (¼ cup) of the coconut milk in a high-speed blender and blend until thick, creamy and completely smooth. This can take a while and you may need to stop frequently to mix the ingredients and push down with your blender's tamper to achieve a smooth consistency. Add extra milk to thin if needed (avoid adding too much extra milk as this is meant to be a thick, soft-serve consistency).

2. Spoon into serving bowls, scatter with the chopped pistachios and serve immediately.

Charlotte's notes

• To present this treat like old-fashioned soft serve, spoon the mixture into a piping bag fitted with a star-shaped nozzle and pipe into serving bowls. Once you have filled the piping bag, put it in the freezer for 5 minutes to allow the soft serve to firm up a little before piping.
• If you plan on making soft serve regularly, keep a batch of ripe frozen banana and avocado in the freezer for convenience. When you have some ripe bananas, peel and chop them into 1.5cm (½ inch) thick slices (one banana cuts into 10–15 slices). Spread the slices out on a baking tray lined with parchment paper and freeze overnight. When frozen place the slices in a freezer-proof container and keep in the freezer until needed. Do the same with the avocado: peel and stone, then cut into 1.5cm (½ inch) cubes (one avocado cuts into 16 cubes) before freezing as above. You will also need these for the smoothies (pages 138–139).

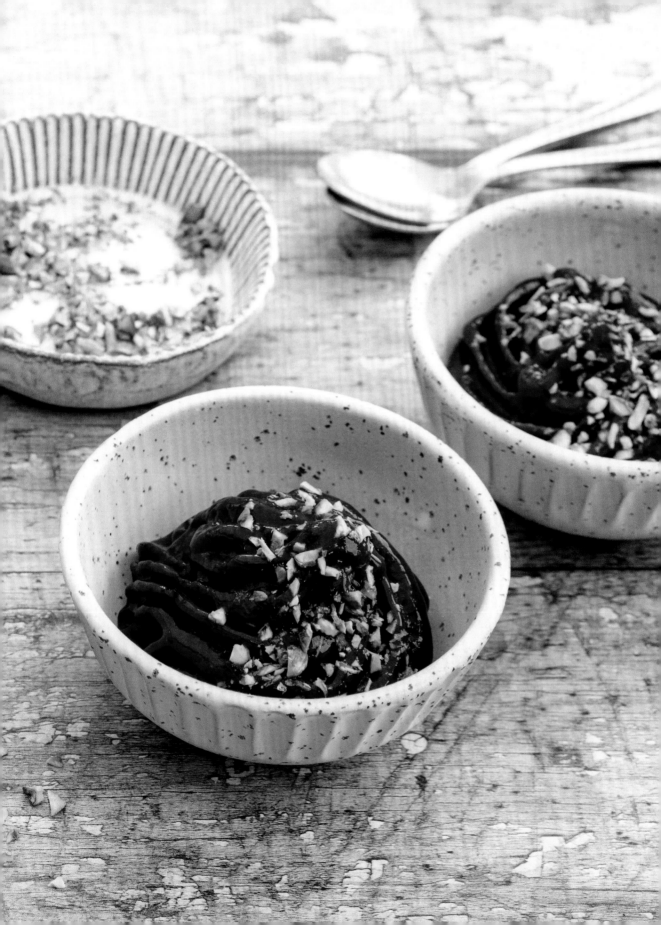

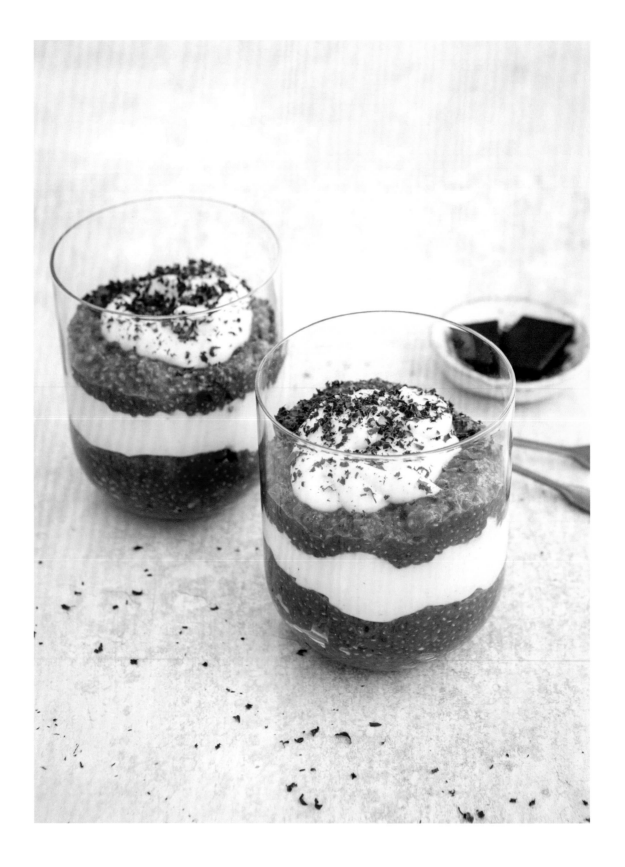

Tiramisu chia puddings

This incredible treat is packed with chocolate and creamy coconut yoghurt and has a rich coffee flavour. It tastes sinful, but it's not!

Serves 2

180ml (¾ cup) almond milk (to make your own, see page 137)
60ml (¼ cup) coconut milk, from a can (to make your own, see page 137)
1 scoop (12g) of coffee protein powder (see notes)
2 tsp cacao powder, sifted
45g (¼ cup) white chia seeds
2 tsp honey
1 tsp vanilla extract
Vanilla coconut yoghurt, to serve
2 squares (20g) dark chocolate (90% cocoa solids), grated, to serve

1. Place the almond milk, coconut milk, coffee protein powder and cacao powder in a blender and blend until smooth. Transfer to a sealable glass container.

2. Add the chia seeds, honey and vanilla extract and whisk to combine. Cover and place in the fridge for at least 4 hours or overnight (the longer you chill the pudding the thicker it becomes).

3. Layer the chia pudding into jam jars, alternating with coconut yoghurt. Finish with a layer of coconut yoghurt, so that you have a total of four layers. Sprinkle with the grated chocolate to serve.

Charlotte's notes

I use Nuzest coffee protein powder, which is caffeine free (see Resources on page 235).

MASTER THE ART

GUT-LOVIN' GUMMIES

An easy way to include gut-healing nutrition,
these gummies couldn't be simpler to make.
If you're hooked on sweets, these will help you
make the transition to a lower-sugar way of life.

The formula

Frozen fruit or fresh juice

- 125g (1 cup) frozen fruit of choice,
  thawed slightly

or

- 250ml (1 cup) pure fruit juice of
  choice

Gelling agent

- 45g (¼ cup) grass-fed
  gelatine (see Resources
  on page 235)

Liquid

- 125ml (½ cup) filtered water or
  coconut water

+

- 60ml (¼ cup) fresh lemon or
  lime juice

Sweetener (try without!)

- 1 tbsp honey or pure
  maple syrup

Makes 20–25 gummies

Watermelon lemon

250ml (1 cup) watermelon juice
125ml (½ cup) coconut water or filtered water
60ml (¼ cup) lemon juice
  (about 2 medium lemons)
45g (¼ cup) grass-fed gelatine
1 tbsp honey (optional)

Mango lime

125g (1 cup) frozen mango, thawed slightly
125ml (½ cup) coconut water or filtered water
60ml (¼ cup) lime juice (about 2 large limes)
Zest of 1 lime
45g (¼ cup) grass-fed gelatine
1 tbsp honey (optional)

Blueberry lemon

125g (1 cup) frozen blueberries, thawed
  slightly
125ml (½ cup) coconut water or filtered water
60ml (¼ cup) lemon juice
  (about 2 medium lemons)
45g (¼ cup) grass-fed gelatine
1 tbsp honey (optional)

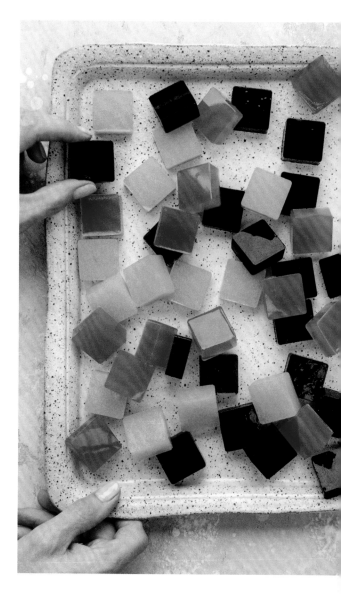

1. Place all the ingredients, except the gelatine and honey, into a blender and blend until smooth.

2. Pour into a small saucepan and sprinkle the gelatine evenly over the top of the mixture and set aside for 5 minutes. It will thicken as the gelatine absorbs the liquid.

3. Place the saucepan over a low heat, add the honey (if using) and whisk gently for 5 minutes, or until smooth and thin.

4. Pour the mixture into silicone square moulds, place on a baking tray and refrigerate overnight, or for at least 2 hours to firm up. Remove from the moulds and store in an airtight glass container in the fridge.

Anti-inflammatory golden milk

Make this deliciously warming golden milk part of your evening ritual. The ultimate soothing drink.

Serves 1

125ml (½ cup) cashew milk (to make your own, see page 137)
125ml (½ cup) oat milk (to make your own, see page 137)
1 serving of collagen powder (see notes)
½ tsp ground turmeric
¼ tsp ground cinnamon
Pinch of ground ginger
Pinch of ground cardamom
1 tsp manuka honey

Place the milks, collagen powder, spices and honey in a blender and blend until smooth and creamy. Pour into a small saucepan set over a low heat for 4–5 minutes, or until warmed through.

Charlotte's notes

• I find that a mix of cashew and oat milks makes the creamiest drink. You can use just one type of milk if you prefer.
• I recommend hydrolysed (easier to absorb) collagen powder (see Resources on page 235).

Revitalising matcha latte

If you love matcha latte but don't want the sugar hit,
try this guilt-free recipe and enjoy an all-natural version
that still tastes delicious.

Serves 1

250ml (1 cup) coconut milk (see notes)
½ tsp manuka honey
1g matcha green tea powder (see Pantry staples on page 90)
½ tsp pure vanilla extract
35g (¼ cup) raw cashews, soaked, drained and rinsed (see notes)

Place the coconut milk, honey, matcha green tea powder, vanilla extract
and cashews in a blender and blend until completely smooth. Pour into
a small saucepan and place over a low heat for 4–5 minutes, or until
warmed through.

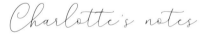

Charlotte's notes

• Use thinner coconut milk from a carton (see Pantry staples
on page 86) rather than coconut milk from a can. To make
your own, see page 137.
• Soak the cashews in twice the volume of filtered water for
at least 2 hours, then drain and rinse thoroughly. The
cashews add a creamy, frothy texture to this latte and are
worth the extra effort.
• There is typically 30mg caffeine per 1g serving of matcha.
See page 71 for more information on caffeine.

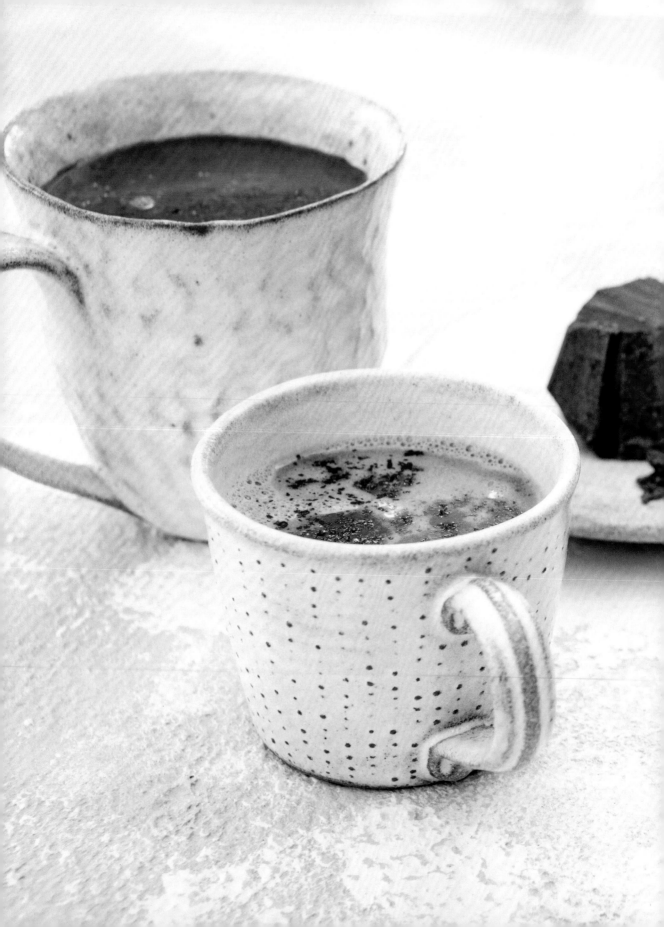

Adaptogenic cinnamon-chai hot chocolate

This hot chocolate is deliciously creamy. With the addition of maca and ashwagandha to aid inner calm and sleep, it's the perfect after-dinner treat.

Serves 1

250ml (1 cup) oat milk (to make your own, see page 137)

1 serving collagen powder (see Resources on page 235)

2 tsp cacao powder, sifted

1 tsp gelatinised maca root powder, sifted (see notes)

½ tsp chai spices, sifted (see Pantry staples on page 84)

½ tsp ground cinnamon, sifted

½ tsp manuka honey (optional)

1 tsp ashwagandha tincture (see notes)

1 tsp light (hulled) tahini

1 tsp finely grated ceremonial grade cacao (see Pantry staples on page 85) or dark chocolate (90% cocoa solids)

1. Place the oat milk, powders, chai spices, cinnamon, honey (if using), ashwagandha tincture and tahini in a blender and blend until completely smooth.

2. Transfer to a saucepan, place over a low heat and simmer for 4–5 minutes, or until warmed through. Pour into a mug and sprinkle with the grated cacao (or chocolate).

Charlotte's notes

• I highly recommend including the collagen powder for two reasons. First, the collagen adds a delicious creaminess to the drink – and who doesn't love a creamy hot chocolate? Second, collagen is one of the richest sources of glycine. Glycine is a conditionally essential amino acid that becomes essential in pregnancy, meaning you must obtain it from your diet.

• For maca powder and ashwagandha, see adaptogens in Resources on page 235.

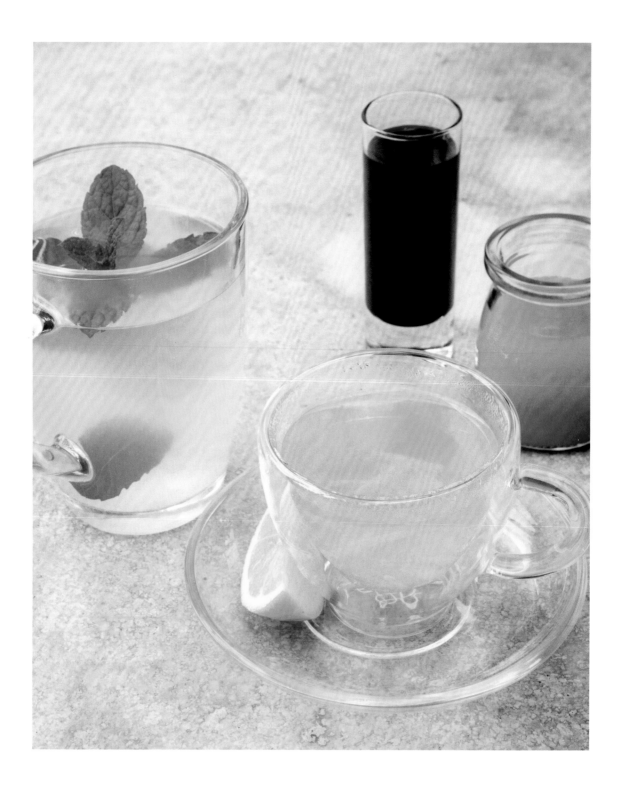

Teas and tonics

A selection of homemade teas and tonics to support your health and vitality.

Start-the-day tea

Serves 1

250ml (1 cup) filtered hot water
Juice of 1 lemon
2 sprigs of mint

Place the water, lemon juice and mint in a teapot. Steep for 5 minutes, then strain into a cup.

Digestive soother

Serves 1

250ml (1 cup) filtered water
2.5cm (1 inch) piece of ginger, peeled and thinly sliced
Juice of 1 lemon
1/4 tsp ground turmeric, sifted
Lemon wedge

Place the water, ginger, lemon juice and turmeric in a small saucepan over a high heat. Bring to a boil, then turn off the heat and steep for 5 minutes. Strain into a cup and add a lemon wedge to serve.

Liver tonic

Serves 1

1 medium beetroot, peeled and chopped
2.5cm (1 inch) piece of ginger
1 tsp lemon juice
Pinch of ground cinnamon

Juice the beetroot and ginger, then whisk in the lemon juice and cinnamon. Pour into a glass and drink as a shot.

Immune tonic

Serves 1

Juice of 1 lemon
Pinch of cayenne pepper
1 tsp grated ginger
1 tsp grated turmeric
20ml (1/8 cup) filtered water

Place the lemon juice, cayenne, ginger, turmeric and water in a small jug and whisk to combine. Pour into a glass and drink as a shot.

Appendix

Guide to soaking and cooking legumes and wholegrains

How to soak and cook legumes

1. Place the legumes in a sieve or colander and rinse thoroughly under running water, then transfer to a large bowl and cover with recently boiled filtered water.

2. Add 2 tablespoons of lemon juice or apple cider vinegar and leave to soak (see table for soaking time).

3. Drain and rinse thoroughly and place in a large saucepan. Cover with filtered water (the water should reach 5cm above the legumes), add a strip of kombu (see Resources, pages 233 and 234). Cover and bring to the boil, skimming off any foam that rises to the top. Reduce the heat and simmer until the beans are tender (see table for cooking time).

4. Once cooked, drain and rinse the legumes and discard the kombu.

The table below indicates the different soaking and cooking times required.

Dried legume	Soaking time	Cooking time (after soaking)
Adzuki beans	At least 1–2 hours	30 minutes
Black beans	Overnight	45–60 minutes
Butter beans	Overnight	60–90 minutes
Chickpeas	Overnight	90 minutes
Kidney beans	Overnight	60 minutes
Lentils, brown/green	At least 1–2 hours	15–20 minutes
Lentils, Puy	At least 1–2 hours	10–15 minutes
Lentils, red	At least 1–2 hours	10–15 minutes
Mung beans	At least 1–2 hours	60 minutes
Pinto beans	Overnight	45–60 minutes
Split peas	At least 1–2 hours	20–30 minutes

Dried grain	Soaking time	Cooking time (after soaking)
Amaranth	At least 6 hours	20 minutes
Buckwheat	At least 2 hours	5–10 minutes
Millet	At least 6 hours	10 minutes
Quinoa	2 hours	15 minutes
Rice, brown	2–4 hours	15 minutes
Rice, wild	At least 4 hours	30 minutes

How to soak and cook grains

1. Place the grains in a sieve or colander and rinse thoroughly under running water until the water runs clear. You can rub the grains together with your hands to help the process. Drain well.

2. Place the grains in a large bowl and cover with warm filtered water. Add 1 tablespoon of lemon juice or apple cider vinegar and leave to soak (see table for soaking time). Drain and rinse thoroughly.

3. Place in a large saucepan and add one and a half times as much filtered water as the volume of the grain and ½ teaspoon of sea salt for every cup of grain. Cover and bring to the boil. Reduce the heat and simmer until the grains are tender and the water is absorbed (see table for cooking time). Do not stir the grains while cooking as this interferes with the cooking process.

4. Remove from the heat and leave the grains to sit for 5 minutes with the lid on. Fluff with a fork before serving.

The table above indicates the different soaking and cooking times required.

Charlotte's notes

• Cooking times may vary, depending on the quality or age of your legumes and grains.
• Use a pressure cooker or Instant Pot for drastically reduced cooking times.
• Some recipes may not recommend soaking lentils and split peas. However, I always recommend doing so because it helps support digestion and reduces the cooking time.
• I recommend batch cooking legumes and grains and freezing in smaller portions so that you have them ready for use during the week for quick meals.

Sugar's many disguises

Read food labels and familiarise yourself with words that mean sugar (there are over 70!):

Agave nectar
Barbados sugar
Barley malt
Beet sugar
Birch syrup
Blackstrap molasses
Brown rice syrup
Brown sugar
Buttered sugar
Buttered syrup
Cane juice
Cane juice crystals
Cane sugar
Caramel
Carob syrup
Castor sugar
Coconut sugar
Coconut syrup
Confectioner's sugar
Corn sweetener
Corn syrup
Corn syrup solids
Crystalline fructose
Date sugar
Date syrup
Demerara sugar
Dextran

Dextrin
Dextrose
Diastatic malt
Diatase
D-ribose
Ethyl malt
Evaporated cane juice
Florida crystals
Fructose
Fruit juice
Fruit juice concentrate
Galactose
Golden sugar
Golden syrup
Grape sugar
Glucose
Glucose solids
High-fructose corn syrup
Honey
Icing sugar
Invert sugar
Lactose
Malt syrup
Maltodextrin
Maltose
Maple syrup
Molasses

Molasses syrup
Muscovado sugar
Oanocha
Oat syrup
Organic raw sugar
Panela sugar
Rapadura
Raw sugar
Refiner's syrup
Rice bran syrup
Rice syrup
Sorghum syrup
Sucanat
Sucrose
Sugar
Sugar beets
Sugar beet syrup
Syrup
Table sugar
Tapioca syrup
Treacle
Treacle sugar
Turbinado sugar
Yellow sugar

Resources

The Fertility Kitchen

Book downloads
www.thefertilitykitchen.co.uk/book-bonuses

The Fertility Kitchen
www.thefertilitykitchen.co.uk

The Fertility Kitchen Community
www.facebook.com/groups/thefertilitykitchen

Apps

Fertility advice, information and support
Fertility Circle

Meditation
Calm
Headspace

Safety profiles of skin care
Think Dirty

Home and personal care

Blue-light-blocking products
Blue Light Glasses
Ocushield

Castor oil packs
Castorvida

Deodorant
Wild

Food wrap and parchment
If You Care
The Beeswax Wrap Co

Hand sanitiser
Neal's Yard Remedies

Health and fitness tracker
Oura

Household products
Bower Collective
EcoVibe
Greenscents
Little Beau Sheep
 (for wool dryer balls)
Seep
Smol

Reusable cups, water bottles and food storage
Black & Blum
Circular & Co
Kilner
Klean Kanteen
Weck

Skincare and makeup
Fushi
Jones Road
RMS Beauty
Vapour Beauty
Votary
Weleda

Ingredients and suppliers

Abel & Cole
For organic vegetables, broccoli sprouts, meat, poultry, eggs and fish

Atlantic Kitchen
For seaweed such as dulse and wakame

Biona Organic (available from Amazon and Ocado)
For coconut aminos, coconut oil, legumes and passata rustica in glass jars

Clearspring
For Japanese foods such as kombu seaweed, mirin, miso paste and tamari

Coconut Merchant
For coconut chips (flakes)

COCOS
For organic, dairy-free coconut yoghurt

Cool Chile Company
For chipotle in adobo smoky paste

Delouis (available from Abel & Cole)
For Dijon mustard

Eaten Alive
For smoked sriracha sauce

Hodmedod's
For British-grown dried beans, legumes and grains

Lalani & Co
For matcha gold green tea powder

Leap Wild
For wild cod and wild sockeye salmon

Linwoods
For sprouted milled flaxseeds (linseeds), and mixed milled flaxseed, pumpkin and sunflower seeds

Monjardin (available from Ocado)
For organic legumes in glass jars

Moulins Mahjoub (available from Abel & Cole)
For artichoke leaves and capers

Mr Organic
For grilled artichokes, passata rustica and toasted sesame oil in glass jars

Nutural World
For coconut cream and nut butters in glass jars

Ossa
For organic, grass-fed ghee and bone broth in glass jars

Plenish
For plant milks

Pure wines
For organic and sulphite-free wines

Real Food Source
For cacao products, coconut products, dried beans and legumes, dried fruits (e.g. banana chips and dates), gluten-free flours (e.g. buckwheat and oat flour), grains (e.g. buckwheat, oats, quinoa and quinoa flakes), nuts and nut butters, powders (e.g. wild blueberry), psyllium husk and seeds

Rebel Kitchen
For raw coconut water

Riverford
For organic vegetables, meat, poultry and eggs

Seedlip
For non-alcoholic spirits

Shipton Mill
For organic gluten-free flours and aluminium-free, gluten-free baking powder

Sky sprouts
For broccoli sprouts

Steenbergs
For extracts, herbs and spices such as Aleppo pepper, brown mustard seeds, chilli flakes and powder, chipotle chillies, ground cinnamon, fennel seeds, garlic powder, Mexican chilli powder blend, onion powder, pilau seasoning blend, Thai spice seasoning, ground turmeric and za'atar

Suma (available from Steenbergs)
For organic light tahini

The Cornish Seaweed Company
For kombu seaweed

The Cultured Collective
For raw sauerkraut and kimchi

The Garlic Farm
For garlic salt

Tiana (available from Amazon and Ocado)
For cassava flour

Supplements

Adaptogens
Fushi
Pukka Herbs

Bone broth
Ossa

Collagen powder
Ancient + Brave
Bare Biology

Fish oil
Bare Biology

Gelatinised maca powder
Gaia Herbs
Vivo Life

Grass-fed pure gelatine powder
Planet Paleo

Medicinal mushrooms
Four Sigmatic
Hifas Da Terra

Protein powder
Form Nutrition
Nuzest

Vitamins and minerals
Allergy Research
Designs For Health
Pure Encapsulations
Seeking Health
Thorne Research
Zooki

Websites

Blood testing services
Medichecks
www.medichecks.com
Thriva
www.thriva.co

Consumer guides on cosmetics, household and consumer products, personal-care products and pesticides
Environmental Working Group
www.ewg.org

Fertility support
Fertility Network UK
www.fertilitynetworkuk.org

Pregnancy and baby loss support
The Worst Girl Gang Ever
www.theworstgirlgangever. co.uk
Tommy's
www.tommys.org

Registered UK nutritional therapists
British Association for Nutrition and Lifestyle Medicine: BANT
www.bant.org.uk

References

For a complete list of references, visit www.thefertilitykitchen.co.uk/book-bonuses.

Page 14

Boots CE, Jungheim ES. Inflammation and Human Ovarian Follicular Dynamics. *Semin Reprod Med*. 2015. doi:10.1055/s-0035-1554928.

Calleja-Agius J, et al. Investigation of systemic inflammatory response in first trimester pregnancy failure. *Hum Reprod*. 2011. doi: 10.1093/humrep/der402.

González F. Inflammation in Polycystic Ovary Syndrome: Underpinning of insulin resistance and ovarian dysfunction. *Steroids*. 2012. doi:10.1016/j.steroids.2011.12.003.

Lin YH. Chronic Niche Inflammation in Endometriosis-Associated Infertility: Current Understanding and Future Therapeutic Strategies. *Int J Mol Sci*. 2018. doi: 10.3390/ijms19082385.

Page 15

Carp HJA, Selmi C, Shoenfeld Y. The autoimmune bases of infertility and pregnancy loss. *J. Autoimmun*. 2012. doi: 10.1016/j.jaut.2011.11.016.

Ghadir M. et al. Unexplained infertility as primary presentation of celiac disease, a case report and literature review. *Iran J Reprod Med*. 2011. PMC4216449.

Jatzko B, et al. The impact of thyroid function on intrauterine insemination outcome - a retrospective analysis. *Reprod Biol Endocrinol*. 2014. doi: 10.1186/1477-7827-12-28.

Martinelli P. Coeliac disease and unfavourable outcome of pregnancy. *Gut*. 2000. doi: 10.1136/gut.46.3.332

Shigesi N, et al. The association between endometriosis and autoimmune diseases: a systematic review and meta-analysis. *Hum Reprod Update*. 2019. doi: 10.1136/gut.46.3.332

Stagnaro-Green A. Thyroid Antibodies and Miscarriage: Where Are We at a Generation Later? *J Thyroid Res* .2011. doi: 10.4061/2011/841949

Page 16

The Institute for Functional Medicine. *This video introduction to the 5R framework for treating digestive disorders is presented by Vincent Pedre, MD*. Available at: https://www.ifm.org/news-insights/5r-framework-gut-health/. Accessed 8 March 2021.

Page 18

Chavarro JE, et al. A prospective study of dairy foods intake and anovulatory infertility. *Hum Reprod*. 2007. doi: 10.1093/humrep/dem019.

Page 32

Jatzko B, et al. The impact of thyroid function on intrauterine insemination outcome - a retrospective analysis. *Reprod Bio Endocrinol*. 2014. doi: 10.1186/1477-7827-12-28.

Orouji Jokar T, et al. Higher TSH Levels Within the Normal Range Are Associated With Unexplained Infertility. *J Clin Endocrinol Metab*. 2017. doi: 10.1210/jc.2017-02120.

Peyneau M, et al. Role of thyroid dysimmunity and thyroid hormones in endometriosis. *PNAS*. 2019. doi: 10.1073/pnas.1820469116.

Poppe K,. et al. Thyroid Dysfunction and Autoimmunity in Infertile Women. *Thyroid*. 2002. doi: 10.1089/105072502320908330.

Poppe K, Velkeniers B, Glinoer D. The role of thyroid autoimmunity in fertility and pregnancy. *Nat Clin Pract Endocrinol Metab*. 2008. doi: 10.1038/ncpendmeto846.

Poppe K, Velkeniers B. Thyroid disorders in infertile women. https://pubmed.ncbi.nlm.nih.gov/12707633/ Accessed 9 April 2021.

Singla R. et al. Thyroid disorders and polycystic ovary syndrome: An emerging relationship. *Indian J Endocrinol Metab*. 2015. doi: 10.4103/2230-8210.14686

Verma I, et al. Prevalence of hypothyroidism in infertile women and evaluation of response of treatment for hypothyroidism on infertility. *Int J App Basic Med Res*. 2012. doi: 10.4103/2230-8210.159058

Page 33

Green KA, et al. Investigating the optimal preconception TSH range for patients undergoing IVF when controlling for embryo quality. *J Assist Reprod Genet*. 2015. doi: 10.1007/s10815-015-0549-4

Page 35

Bajaj JK. Various Possible Toxicants Involved in Thyroid Dysfunction: A Review. *J Clin Diagn Res*. 2016. doi: 10.7860/JCDR/2016/15195.7092

Diamanti-Kandarakis E, et al. Endocrine-Disrupting Chemicals: An Endocrine Society Scientific Statement. *Endocr Revs*. 2009. doi: 10.1210/er.2009-0002

Lee JE, Choi K. Perfluoroalkyl substances exposure and thyroid hormones in humans: epidemiological observations and implications. *Ann Pediatr Endocrinol Metab*. 2017. doi: 10.6065/apem.2017.22.1.6.

Page 36

Franks S, Hardy K. Androgen Action in the Ovary. *Front Endocrinol*. 2018. doi: 10.3389/fendo.2018.00452

Lebbe M, Woodruff TK. Involvement of androgens in ovarian health and disease. *Mol Hum Reprod*. 2013. Doi: 10.1093/molehr/gato65.

Prizant H, Gleicher N, Sen A. Androgen actions in the ovary: balance is key. *J Endocrinol*. 2014. doi: 10.1530/JOE-14-0296

Page 37

Butts S, et al. Correlation of telomere length and telomerase activity with occult ovarian insufficiency. *J Clinl Endocrinol and Metab*. 2009. doi: 10.1210/jc.2008-2269

Hanna CW. et al. Telomere length and reproductive aging. *Hum Reprod*, 2009. doi: 10.1093/humrep/dep007.

Kalmbach K, et al. Telomeres and Female Reproductive Aging. *Sem Reprod Med*. 2015. doi: 10.1055/s-0035-1567823.

Keefe DL, et al. Telomere length predicts embryo fragmentation after in vitro fertilization in women--toward a telomere theory of reproductive aging in women. *Am J Obstet Gynecol*. 2005. doi: 10.1016/j.ajog.2005.01.036

Keefe DL, Liu L, Marquard K. Telomeres and meiosis in health and disease. *Cell Mol Life Sci*. 2007. doi: 10.1007/s00018-006-6462-3.

Treff NR, et al. Telomere DNA Deficiency Is Associated with Development of Human Embryonic Aneuploidy. *PLoS Genet*, 2011. doi: 10.1371/journal.pgen.1002161.

Vasilopoulos E, et al. The association of female and male infertility with telomere length (Review). *Intl J Mol Med*. 2019. doi: 10.3892/ijmm.2019.4225.

Page 40

Czeczuga-Semeniuk E, Wolczynski S. identification of carotenoids in ovarian tissue in women. https://pubmed.ncbi.nlm.nih.gov/16211314/ Accessed 9 May 2021.

Page 41
Agarwal A, Allamaneni SSR. Sperm DNA damage assessment: a test whose time has come. *Fertil Steril*, 2005, doi: 10.1016/j.fertnstert.2005.03.080
Virro MR, Larson-Cook KL, Evenson DP. Sperm chromatin structure assay (scsa®) parameters are related to fertilization, blastocyst development, and ongoing pregnancy in in vitro fertilization and intracytoplasmic sperm injection cycles. *Fertil Steril*, 2004. doi: 10.1016/j.fertnstert.2003.09.063.

Page 42
Durairajanayagam D. Lifestyle causes of male infertility. *Arab J Urol*. 2018. doi: 10.1016/j.aju.2017.12.004

Page 43
Janevic T, et al. Effects of work and life stress on semen quality. *Fertil Steril*. 2014. doi: 10.1016/j.fertnstert.2014.04.021
Li Y et al. Association between socio-psycho-behavioral factors and male semen quality: systematic review and meta-analyses. *Fertil Steril*. 2011. doi: 10.1016/j.fertnstert.2010.06.031.
Nargund VH. Effects of psychological stress on male fertility. *Nat Rev Urol*. 2015. doi: 10.1038/nrurol.2015.112.
Stone BA, et al. Age thresholds for changes in semen parameters in men. *Fertil Steril*. 2013. Doi: 10.1016/j.fertnstert.2013.05.046.

Page 44
Ricci E, et al. Coffee and caffeine intake and male infertility: a systematic review. *Nutr J*. 2017. doi: 10.1186/s12937-017-0257-2.

Page 45
Ahmadi S, et al. Antioxidant supplements and semen parameters: An evidence based review. *Intl J Reprod Biomed*. 2016. PMC5203687.

Page 46
Salas-Huetos A, et al. Effect of nut consumption on semen quality and functionality in healthy men consuming a Western-style diet: a randomized controlled trial. *Am J Clin Nutr*. 2018. doi: 10.1093/ajcn/nqy181.

Page 50
Environmental Working Group. *EWG's 2019 Shopper's Guide to Pesticides in ProduceTM*, Available at: https://www.ewg.org/foodnews/summary.php. Accessed 10 May 2021.

Page 59
Gaskins AJ, et al. Seafood Intake, Sexual Activity, and Time to Pregnancy. *J Clin Endocrinol Metab*. 2018. doi: 10.1210/jc.2018-00385.

Page 61
Elango R, Ball RO. Protein and Amino Acid Requirements during Pregnancy. *Adv Nutr*. 2016. doi: 10.3945/an.115.011817.

Page 62
Chiu YH. et al. Serum omega-3 fatty acids and treatment outcomes among women undergoing assisted reproduction. *Hum Reprod*. 2017. doi: 10.1093/humrep/dex335.
Hammiche F, et al. Increased preconception omega-3 polyunsaturated fatty acid intake improves embryo morphology. *Fertil Steril*. 2011. doi: 10.1016/j.fertnstert.2010.11.021.
Matorras R, et al. Fatty acid composition of fertilization-failed human oocytes. *Hum Reprod*. 1998. doi: 10.1093/humrep/13.8.2227.
Moran L, et al. Altered Preconception Fatty Acid Intake Is Associated with Improved Pregnancy Rates in Overweight and Obese Women Undertaking in Vitro Fertilisation. *Nutrients*, 2016. doi: 10.3390/nu8010010.

Page 71
Chen LW, et al. Maternal caffeine intake during pregnancy and risk of pregnancy loss: a categorical and dose–response meta-analysis of prospective studies. *Public Health Nutr*, 2015. doi: 10.1017/S1368980015002463.
Gaskins AJ, et al. Pre-pregnancy caffeine and caffeinated beverage intake and risk of spontaneous abortion. *Eur J f Nutr*, 2016. doi: 10.1007/s00394-016-1301-2

Page 80
Dawodu A, et al. Randomized Controlled Trial (RCT) of Vitamin D Supplementation in Pregnancy in a Population With Endemic Vitamin D Deficiency. *J Clin Endocrinol Metab*, 2013. doi: 10.1210/jc.2013-1154.
Dunstan JA, et al. Cognitive assessment of children at age 21/2 years after maternal fish oil supplementation in pregnancy: a randomised controlled trial. *Arch Dis Child Fetal Neonatal Ed*, 2008. doi: 10.1136/adc.2006.099085.
Helland IB, et al. Maternal Supplementation With Very-Long-Chain n-3 Fatty Acids During Pregnancy and Lactation Augments Children's IQ at 4 Years of Age. *Pediatr*, 2003. doi: 10.1542/peds.111.1.e39
Jiang X, et al. A higher maternal choline intake among third-trimester pregnant women lowers placental and circulating concentrations of the antiangiogenic factor fms-like tyrosine kinase-1 (sFLT1). *FASEB J*, 2013. doi: 10.1096/fj.12-221648
Jiang X, et al. Maternal choline intake alters the epigenetic state of fetal cortisol-regulating genes in humans. *FASEB J*. 2012. doi: 10.7860/JCDR/2016/15195.7092

Page 107
Nedergaard M, Goldman SA. Brain Drain. *SciAm*. 2016. doi: 10.1258/jrsm.98.11.487.

Page 108
Tamura H, et al. The role of melatonin as an antioxidant in the follicle. *J Ovarian Res*. 2012. doi: 10.1186/1757-2215-5-5.

Page 111
Speed C. Exercise and menstrual function. *BMJ*, 2007. doi: 10.1136/bmj.39043.625498.80.

Page 113
Diamanti-Kandarakis E, et al. Endocrine-Disrupting Chemicals: An Endocrine Society Scientific Statement. *Endocr Revs*. 2009. doi: 10.1210/er.2009-0002
Karwacka A, et al. Exposure to modern, widespread environmental endocrine disrupting chemicals and their effect on the reproductive potential of women: an overview of current epidemiological evidence. *Hum Fertil*. 2017. Doi: 10.1080/14647273.2017.1358828.
Knez J. Endocrine-disrupting chemicals and male reproductive health. *Reprod BioMed Online*. 2013. doi: 10.1016/j.rbmo.2013.02.005.

Index

Acknowledgements

Mum and Dad, thank you for instilling in me a strong work ethic and for believing in and supporting me always.

Jeremy, thank you for your unwavering support and for making it possible for me to pursue my dreams. George and Alex, you are my world. Without you, The Fertility Kitchen wouldn't exist. You are incredible and I'm thankful for you every day.

Maria, you have been my rock from the beginning of this process to the end. I appreciate everything you have done for me. Lindsay, Lindsay, Laura, and VJ thank you for your words of wisdom, advice and friendship.

Thank you to Rowan Lawton, my literary agent, and to Jane Sturrock and the Quercus team, for believing in The Fertility Kitchen and for your incredible support and vision. Many thanks also to Corinne Colvin, Tokiko Morishima, Peter Liddiard and Anna Southgate. Thank you to Andrew Hayes-Watkins and Ellie Mulligan for an epic week on the book shoot, I had a blast.

Finally, thank you to my clients and to everyone who has supported me and The Fertility Kitchen. This book is a dream come true and it wouldn't have been possible without you.

Picture credits

Photography Andrew Hayes-Watkins except: Shutterstock ©: pages 30, 40, 43, 46, 47, 49, 50, 52–53, 55, 57, 64, 70, 74, 75, 83, 85, 86, 87, 90, 91, 92, 93, 94, 95, 114.